Food and Drug Interactions

A Guide for Consumers

Gary A. Holt, M.Ed., Ph.D., R.Ph.
Pharmacy Practice, Pharmacy Administration and Public Health

Precept Press, Chicago
A Division of Bonus Books, Inc.

Library of Congress Cataloging-in-Publication Data

Holt, Gary A.
Food and drug interactions : a guide for consumers / Gary A. Holt.
p. cm.
Includes bibliographical references and index.
ISBN 0-944496-59-8
1. Drug-nutrient interactions. I. Title.
RM302.4.H65 1998
615'.7045—dc21 97-37129
CIP

02 01 00 99 98 5 4 3 2 1

Precept Press
Division of Bonus Books, Inc.
160 East Illinois Street
Chicago, Illinois 60611

Printed in the United States of America

Contributors

Ashish Chandra, M.M.S., M.B.A., Ph.D.
Pharmacy Administration

Janis Gulick, M.D.
Clinical Pharmacy

Neil Henann, Pharm.D.
Clinical Pharmacy

Tracy Hunter, Ph.D., R.Ph.
Division Head, Pharmacy Practice

Harvey Rappaport, Ph.D., R.Ph.
Pharmacy Administration and Pharmacy Practice

William H. Ross, B.S., R.Ph.
Clinical Pharmacy and Drug Information

James Talley, M.S.
Clinical Pharmacy

Contributors to First Edition

Robin Ferencik, R.Ph.
Pharmacy Practice

Reed Heflin, M.S., R.Ph.
Pharmacy Practice

Helen Lini, R.Ph.
Pharmacy Practice

Lori Nelson-Allen, R.Ph.
Pharmacy Practice

Linda Sutherland, M.B.A., R.Ph.
Drug Information Specialist

Table of Contents

INTRODUCTION ix

USE OF THIS MANUAL xi

FOOD & DRUG INTERACTIONS 1

APPENDICES

1. Nutrient Content of Selected Foods 291
2. Vitamin Content of Selected Foods 299
3. Examples of Foods Containing Selected Nutrients 309
4. Foods that Acidify the Urine 313
5. Foods that Alkalinize the Urine 315
6. Foods Associated with the Development of Headaches 317
7. Foods that Contain Tyramine and other Pressor Amines 319
8. Physiologically and Pharmacologically Active Agents in Foods 321
9. Drugs Associated with Changes in Appetite 323
10. Symptoms Associated with the MAOI Reaction 325
11. Symptoms Associated with the Disulfiram Reaction 327
12. Calcium—Symptoms of Deficiency and Excess 329
13. Folic Acid—Symptoms of Deficiency and Excess 331
14. Iron—Symptoms of Deficiency and Excess 333
15. Magnesium—Symptoms of Deficiency and Excess 335
16. Potassium—Symptoms of Deficiency and Excess 337
17. Sodium—Symptoms of Deficiency and Excess 339
18. Vitamin A—Symptoms of Deficiency and Excess 341
19. Vitamin B_1—Symptoms of Deficiency and Excess 343
20. Vitamin B_2—Symptoms of Deficiency and Excess 345
21. Vitamin B_3—Symptoms of Deficiency and Excess 347
22. Vitamin B_6—Symptoms of Deficiency and Excess 349
23. Vitamin B_{12}—Symptoms of Deficiency and Excess 351
24. Vitamin C—Symptoms of Deficiency and Excess 353
25. Vitamin D—Symptoms of Deficiency and Excess 355
26. Vitamin E—Symptoms of Deficiency and Excess 357
27. Vitamin K—Symptoms of Deficiency and Excess 359
28. Zinc—Symptoms of Deficiency and Excess 361
29. Drug Brand Name Conversion Chart 363

REFERENCES 391

INDEX 401

Introduction

For quite some time there has been a growing interest in the potential interactions that can occur between drugs and foods. The existence of nearly a million drug products and an infinite number of foods creates a bewildering potential for both positive and negative outcomes to occur when certain foods and drugs are taken together.

The present volume is a summary of food and drug interactions that have appeared in articles and references from medical and health literature. Because of variations in wording that occurred from one citation to another, every effort was made to represent the interactions in a manner that accurately reflected the intent of the original citations. The actual clinical significance of any interaction depends upon a variety of potential variables which include the amount of drug and food being consumed, the age, gender and medical status of the patient, and other considerations. Thus, potential interactions must be evaluated with reference to the particular patient scenario involved. Drug/food interactions listed in this project may or may not occur in a given patient depending upon a variety of factors which can be involved in any given patient scenario.

This project is not intended to serve as a substitute for appropriate clinical assessment and judgment regarding therapy of individual patients.

You should always consult a physician or other appropriate health care professional before making changes in your prescribed medical therapy.

The present listing includes some drug agents which are no longer included in contemporary therapeutic regimens. These agents have been included because of their similarity to agents which continue to be used in contemporary medical practice and/or medical research.

Use of this Manual

This book is presented in outline form and summarizes traditional medical and consumer literature sources. Information in each interaction has been consistently organized in the same format in an effort to facilitate use.

No attempt has been made to indicate the significance of the interactions listed. The actual clinical significance can vary depending upon numerous factors, including the amount of drug and food consumed, as well as a variety of patient characteristics (e.g., weight, gender, disease states which exist). These variables should be taken into account when attempting to evaluate possible clinical outcomes.

This book represents a summary of literature sources. It is intended only as a guide, and is not intended to serve as a substitute for clinical expertise and professional judgment.

Because this book was designed as a consumer reference, references were not included with each citation. However, interested readers may contact the authors for specific references for individual listings.

Some agents can be viewed as either foods or drugs (e.g., vitamins, minerals and electrolytes). They are included as a "food" or a "drug" depending primarily upon how they were listed in their original citations. In other cases, they were listed as a "food" when the interaction involved another agent which is only available as a "drug." The index includes a listing of all agents which appear in either the "food" or "drug" heading. This allows for the reader to find all interactions involving a particular agent regardless of how it was listed.

Please note that many of the "foods" (e.g., potassium, zinc, calcium, Vitamin B) are also found in common antacids and vitamin and mineral supplements.

A-1

Drug: **Acarbose**

Food: Food in general

Outcome: Is taken with meals to prevent absorption of carbohydrates and results in a smaller rise in blood sugar levels after eating.

What to Do: Take acarbose at the start (with the first bite) of your main meals.

A-2

Drug: **ACE Inhibitors**

Food: Potassium

Outcome: Potassium retention is possible.

What to Do: Eat a balanced diet. Your doctor will recommend dietary restrictions if they are indicated. Report any unusual symptoms (see Appendix 16) to your doctor, nurse or pharmacist.

A-3

Drug: **Acetaminophen**

Food: Alcohol

Outcome: Alcohol can increase the risk of acetaminophen toxicity (liver damage). The risk is increased with excessive or chronic use of alcohol.

What to Do: It is best to avoid taking alcohol and acetaminophen together. The drug is especially risky for alcoholics who already have signs of liver damage (e.g., jaundice, low blood sugar) or for heavy drinkers.

A-4

Drug: **Acetaminophen**

Food: Cabbage, brussels sprouts, cruciferous vegetables (large amounts)

Outcome: These foods may interfere with the absorption of acetaminophen, although the overall effectiveness of therapy may not be significantly affected. It has also been reported that these foods may increase the metabolism and elimination of the drug. It is possible that the drug might not work as effectively as usual.

What to Do: If the drug does not appear to be working, check with your doctor, nurse or pharmacist.

A-5

Drug: **Acetaminophen**

Food: Food in general, foods high in pectins, carbohydrates, dates, crackers, jellies

Outcome: These foods may interfere with the absorption of acetaminophen, although the overall effectiveness of therapy may not be significantly affected. It is possible that the drug might not work as effectively as usual.

What to Do: If the drug does not appear to be working, check with your doctor, nurse or pharmacist.

A-6

Drug: **Acetazolamide**

Food: Foods that acidify the urine (see Appendix 4)

Outcome: Your body may not be able to eliminate acetazolamide normally; the effects of the drug can be prolonged and exaggerated.

What to Do: Eat a balanced diet. This interaction is unlikely unless you are consuming large amounts of these foods. Your doctor will recommend dietary changes if they are indicated. If you experience unusual side effects or other symptoms, contact your doctor, nurse or pharmacist.

A-7

Drug: **Acetazolamide**

Food: Foods that produce alkaline urine (see Appendix 5)

Outcome: Acetazolamide may be eliminated from the body more quickly than usual.

What to Do: Eat a balanced diet. This interaction is unlikely unless you are consuming large amounts of these foods. Your doctor will recommend dietary changes if they are indicated. If it seems that the drug is not working, contact your doctor, nurse or pharmacist.

A-8

Drug: **Adrenal Corticosteroids**

Food: Calcium

Outcome: Corticosteroids can interfere with vitamin D activity and inhibit calcium absorption.

What to Do: If corticosteroids are to be taken over a long time period, talk with a health professional about the potential need for calcium supplements. Report any unusual symptoms (see Appendices 17, 27) to your doctor, nurse or pharmacist.

A-9

Drug: **Adrenal Corticosteroids**

Food: Food in general, sodium

Outcome: Fluid and electrolyte disturbances, changes in nitrogen levels, protein breakdown and redistribution of body fat can occur when corticosteroids are taken for long periods of time.

What to Do: Eat a healthy diet, including low fat intake. Your doctor will recommend dietary changes or supplements if they are indicated. Report any unusual symptoms to your doctor, nurse or pharmacist.

A-10

Drug: **Adrenal Corticosteroids**

Food: Vitamin D

Outcome: Corticosteroids can interfere with normal vitamin D activity, which in turn, can inhibit calcium absorption.

What to Do: Eat a healthy diet, including adequate calcium intake. Your doctor may recommend calcium supplements and other dietary changes. Be sure to keep all appointments with your doctor. Report any unusual symptoms (see Appendices 12, 25) to your doctor, nurse or pharmacist.

A-11

Drug: **Alcohol**

Food: Fats, folic acid, magnesium, xylose, methionine, nitrogen, vitamin B_1(thiamine), vitamin B_{12}

Outcome: Long term use of alcohol (especially large amounts) can interfere with the normal absorption of many vitamins, minerals and other nutrients. This can result in various nutrient deficiencies.

What to Do: If you drink heavily, discuss potential health problems with your doctor. It is important to eat a healthy diet. Vitamin and mineral supplementation may be recommended. Discuss this possibility with your doctor, nurse, or pharmacist.

A-12

Drug: **Alcohol**

Food: Food in general

Outcome: Alcohol absorption is reduced when consumed immediately after meals. The overall effect is complex and appears to be related to many factors, including the types and amounts of foods consumed.

What to Do: No interventions are required. In fact, it is usually beneficial to eat before drinking alcoholic beverages.

A-13

Drug: **Alcohol**

Food: Ink caps fungus

Outcome: A disulfiram-type reaction (see Appendix 11) can occur because the fungus is able to interfere with normal alcohol metabolism.

What to Do: Avoid this combination.

A-14

Drug: **Alcohol**

Food: Vitamin A

Outcome: Excessive intake of vitamin A can increase the risk of liver damage by alcohol. A decrease in vitamin A absorption is also possible.

What to Do: If you drink heavily, discuss potential health problems with your doctor. It is important to eat a healthy diet. Your doctor will recommend dietary changes if they are indicated. Report any unusual symptoms (see Appendix 18) to your doctor, nurse or pharmacist.

A-15

Drug: **Alcohol**

Food: Zinc deficient diet

Outcome: It appears that zinc levels affect the ability of the body to metabolize and eliminate alcohol. Alcohol levels may remain higher for longer time periods in patients with zinc-deficient diets.

What to Do: It is always best to drink alcohol in moderation, if you drink at all. If you drink heavily, discuss potential health problems with your doctor. It is important to eat a healthy diet. Your doctor will recommend dietary changes if they are indicated.

A-16

Drug: **Alendronate**

Food: Food in general

Outcome: Food interferes with the absorption of alendronate.

What to Do: Take on an empty stomach (1 hour before or 2 hours after meals) with a full glass of water. Do not eat or drink anything (including orange juice, coffee) so that the drug can work most effectively. Do not recline for 30 minutes following the dose.

A-17

Drug: **Allopurinol**

Food: Diets rich in urates

Outcome: These foods can reduce the effectiveness of allopurinol.

What to Do: Eat a balanced diet. Your doctor will recommend dietary changes if they are indicated. Contact your doctor, nurse or pharmacist if your symptoms are not improving or if you feel that the drug is not working.

A-18

Drug: **Alprazolam**

Food: Alcohol

Outcome: This can be a dangerous mix. It can result in excessive (and possibly dangerous) sedation and depression of the central nervous system (e.g., loss of coordination, impaired judgment, decreased performance skills and alertness, slowed reaction time, increased risk of falls).

What to Do: Avoid this mix. Do not drive, operate machinery or engage in activities that require mental alertness after taking these substances (either alone or in combination). In general, alcohol should be avoided while taking medications of any kind.

A-19

Drug: **Alprazolam**

Food: Caffeine

Outcome: These substances counter each other's effects.

What to Do: It is best to avoid this combination if possible. If alprazolam does not seem to be working effectively, contact your doctor.

A-20

Drug: **Alprazolam**

Food: Food in general

Outcome: Food can interfere with the absorption of many drugs, including alprazolam. However, this interference may not be significant and can vary from one person to another.

What to Do: If alprazolam does not seem to be working effectively, contact your doctor, nurse or pharmacist.

A-21

Drug: **Aluminum Hydroxide**

Food: Calcium, phosphorus, vitamins and minerals.

Outcome: Antacids can interefere with the absorption of many nutrients.

What to Do: Avoid taking antacids and drugs together. Space the dosing by 1-2 hours.

A-22

Drug: **Amiloride**

Food: Potassium (see Appendix 1)

Outcome: Increased potassium levels and activity can occur.

What to Do: Report any unusual symptoms (see Appendix 16) to your doctor or pharmacist.

A-23

Drug: **Aminoglycosides**

Food: Calcium, magnesium, potassium, carbohydrates

Outcome: Decreased levels of certain nutrients have been reported.

What to Do: Antibiotic therapy usually lasts less than 2 weeks, so it is unlikely that this interaction will become a problem. If you are taking antibiotics for long time periods, talk to your doctor, nurse or pharmacist about whether or not nutritional supplements or dietary changes are needed.

A-24

Drug: **Aminoglycosides**

Food: Foods that acidify the urine (see Appendix 4)

Outcome: This combination can interfere with the ability of the body to excrete the drug. So, drug levels, activity and adverse effects can increase.

What to Do: Antibiotic therapy usually lasts less than 2 weeks. Additionally, this interaction would only be expected to occur if large quantities of these food items are being consumed, so it is unlikely that this interaction will become a problem. If you are taking antibiotics for long time periods, talk to your doctor, nurse or pharmacist about whether or not nutritional supplements or dietary changes are needed.

A-25

Drug: **Aminoglycosides**

Food: Foods that produce alkaline urine (see Appendix 5).

Outcome: Alkaline urine can result in a decrease in antibiotic activity.

What to Do: This interaction is unlikely to occur unless you are eating large amounts of these foods. So, it is unlikely that this interaction will become a problem. If you are taking antibiotics for long time periods or if your infection does not seem to be improving, talk to your doctor, nurse or pharmacist about whether or not dietary or therapeutic changes are needed.

A-26

Drug: **Aminoglycosides**

Food: Vitamin A

Outcome: The drug can result in decreased vitamin levels in the body.

What to Do: No interventions are usually necessary, since antibiotic therapy normally lasts less than 2 weeks. Eat a balanced diet. Your doctor will recommend dietary changes if they are necessary. Report unusual symptoms (see Appendix 18) to your doctor, nurse or pharmacist.

A-27

Drug: **Amitriptyline**

Food: Alcohol

Outcome: Increased drug levels, activity and a greater risk of adverse drug effects (e.g., sedation, reduced alertness and reflexes) can occur with this mix. Both alcohol and amitriptyline are sedating. This mix can result in excessive (and possibly dangerous) sedation and depression of the central nervous system (e.g., loss of coordination, impaired judgment, decreased performance skills and alertness, slowed reaction time, increased risk of falls).

What to Do: It is best to avoid this combination. Report unusual symptoms to your doctor, nurse or pharmacist.

A-28

Drug: **Amitriptyline**

Food: Foods that acidify the urine (see Appendix 4)

Outcome: The drug is excreted more quickly than usual in acid urine. This could cause the drug to work less effectively.

What to Do: Eat a balanced diet. This interaction is not likely to be a problem unless you are eating large quantities of these foods while on therapy. If the drug does not seem to be working, contact your doctor, nurse or pharmacist.

A-29

Drug: **Amitriptyline**

Food: Foods that produce alkaline urine (see Appendix 5)

Outcome: The drug is not excreted as quickly as usual in alkaline urine. Drug levels and activity (including adverse drug effects) may increase.

What to Do: Eat a balanced diet. This interaction is not likely to be a problem unless you are eating large quantities of these foods while on therapy. Notify your doctor, nurse or pharmacist if side effects become uncomfortable or if new symptoms appear.

A-30

Drug: **Amitriptyline**

Food: Vitamin C (ascorbic acid)

Outcome: The drug is excreted more quickly than usual in acid urine. This could cause the drug to work less effectively.

What to Do: This interaction is not likely to be a problem unless you are consuming larges quantities of vitamin C while on therapy. If the drug does not seem to be working, contact your doctor, nurse or pharmacist.

A-31

Drug: **Amlodipine**

Food: Grapefruit juice

Outcome: Increased absorption, drug levels and activity (including adverse drug effects) of amlodipine can occur.

What to Do: It is best to take medications with water, rather than other fluids. Report any unusual side effects (e.g., flushing, headache, rapid pulse, hypotension) to your doctor, nurse or pharmacist.

A-32

Drug: **Ammonium Chloride**

Food: Foods that acidify the urine (see Appendix 4)

Outcome: Ammonium chloride is excreted more quickly than usual in acid urine. This could cause the drug to work less effectively.

What to Do: Eat a balanced diet. This interaction is not likely to be a problem unless you are eating large quantities of these foods while on therapy. If the drug does not seem to be working, contact your doctor, nurse or pharmacist.

A-33

Drug: **Ammonium Chloride**

Food: Foods that produce alkaline urine (see Appendix 5)

Outcome: Ammonium chloride is not excreted as quickly as usual in alkaline urine. Its levels and activity (including adverse drug effects) may increase.

What to Do: Eat a balanced diet. This interaction is not likely to be a problem unless you are eating large quantities of these foods while on therapy. Notify your doctor, nurse or pharmacist if side effects become uncomfortable or if new symptoms appear.

A-34

Drug: **Amoxicillin**

Food: Food in general

Outcome: Food delays absorption of the amoxicillin.

What to Do: It is usually best to take antibiotics on an empty stomach (1 hour before or 2 hours after eating). If the drug seems to irritate your stomach (e.g. nausea, vomiting, abdominal pain), take it with a small amount of food. Even though food can delay absorption, it does not usually have a negative impact on therapy. Contact your doctor if you feel that the drug is not working.

A-35

Drug: **Amphetamine**

Food: Foods that acidify the urine (see Appendix 4)

Outcome: Amphetamines are excreted more quickly than usual in acid urine. This could cause them to work less effectively.

What to Do: Eat a balanced diet. This interaction is not likely to be a problem unless you are eating large quantities of these foods while on therapy. If the drug does not seem to be working, contact your doctor, nurse or pharmacist.

A-36

Drug: **Amphetamine**

Food: Foods that produce alkaline urine (see Appendix 5)

Outcome: The drug is not excreted as quickly as usual in alkaline urine. Drug levels and activity (including adverse drug effects) may increase.

What to Do: Eat a balanced diet. This interaction is not likely to be a problem unless you are eating large quantities of these foods while on therapy. Notify your doctor, nurse or pharmacist if side effects become uncomfortable or if new symptoms appear.

A-37

Drug: **Amphetamines**

Food: Vitamin C

Outcome: Increased excretion and decreased effects of amphetamines can occur.

What to Do: It is best to avoid excessive intake of the vitamin. Eat a balanced diet and drink ample water. Consult with your doctor, nurse or pharmacist if your therapy does not seem to be working effectively.

A-38

Drug: **Ampicillin**

Food: Acidic fruit or juices, carbonated beverages, wine, syrups, acidic beverages

Outcome: Acidic beverages can cause ampicillin to decompose prematurely. Antibiotic activity can be reduced.

What to Do: Take antibiotics with water, rather than other fluids.

A-39

Drug: **Ampicillin**

Food: Food in general

Outcome: Food can reduce or delay absorption of ampicillin. This can result in decreased drug levels and activity.

What to Do: It is usually best to take antibiotics on an empty stomach (1 hour before or 2 hours after eating). However, take it with a small amount of food if the drug is irritating to your stomach. Talk with your doctor, nurse or pharmacist if you feel that the drug is not working effectively.

A-40

Drug: **Anabolic Steroids**

Food: Food in general

Outcome: Fluid and electrolyte retention and related problems (e.g., swelling) can occur.

What to Do: Notify your doctor, nurse or pharmacist if you experience unusual symptoms of any kind.

A-41

Drug: **Angina Drugs**

Food: Alcohol

Outcome: Alcohol dilates blood vessels, which can result in drops in blood pressure, dizziness and fainting, especially when arising from a seated or lying position. Also, alcohol can mask pain that normally serves as a warning signal of problems. Long term alcohol use can damage heart muscles.

What to Do: It is best to avoid alcohol if you are being treated for heart problems, high blood pressure or other vascular diseases. Check with your doctor, nurse or pharmacist if you have questions about the use of alcohol with the medications you are taking.

A-42

Drug: **Antacids**

Food: High molecular protein solutions

Outcome: Mixing high molecular protein solution with antacids results in a gelatinous mass that may not be absorbed well.

What to Do: Avoid this mix.

A-43

Drug: **Antacids**

Food: Fluoride, iron, phosphorus, vitamins (e.g., A, B_1, D)

Outcome: Decreased absorption of these nutrients can occur. This can result in deficiencies over time.

What to Do: Avoid taking these nutrients and antacids together. It is best to take antacids 1 hour before or 2 hours after food or nutritional supplements.

A-44

Drug: **Antacids—Aluminum Hydroxide**

Food: Phosphorus, liver, meat, egg yolk, milk, cheese, peanuts, whole-grain cereals

Outcome: Aluminum binds with phosphorus in these foods so that it is not absorbed normally. Potassium loss can cause calcium to be lost from bones. This can result in brittle bones. The risk for problems is especially high for people with chronic kidney failure.

What to Do: Eat a balanced diet. No specific interventions are usually indicated, since antacids should not be used for more than a week without consulting a health professional.

A-45

Drug: **Anti-Anxiety Drugs**

Food: Alcohol

Outcome: This mix can result in excessive (and possibly dangerous) sedation and depression of the central nervous system (e.g., loss of coordination, impaired judgment, decreased performance skills and alertness, slowed reaction time, increased risk of falls).

What to Do: Avoid this mix.

A-46

Drug: **Anti-Arrhythmia Drugs**

Food: Coffee, tea, caffeine

Outcome: Decreased drug effectiveness can occur.

What to Do: It is best to drink decaffeinated beverages. Notify your doctor, nurse or pharmacist if the drug does not appear to be working effectively.

A-47

Drug: **Antibiotics**

Food: Alcohol

Outcome: Headache, stomach cramping, nausea and vomiting can occur.

What to Do: Avoid taking alcohol and antibiotics together.

A-48

Drug: **Antibiotics**

Food: Amino Acids

Outcome: Impaired protein synthesis has been reported.

What to Do: Eat a balanced diet. Antibiotics are usually taken for less than 2 weeks, so it is unlikely that this interaction will cause problems. Your doctor will recommend dietary changes if they are indicated.

A-49

Drug: **Antibiotics**

Food: Calcium

Outcome: Some antibiotics can interfere with calcium absorption.

What to Do: Eat a balanced diet. Antibiotics are usually taken for less than 2 weeks, so it is unlikely that this interaction will cause problems. Your doctor will recommend dietary changes if they are indicated.

A-50

Drug: **Antibiotics**

Food: Food in general

Outcome: Food can reduce or delay absorption of these drugs, which can result in decreased levels and activity of antibiotics.

What to Do: It is usually best to take antibiotics on an empty stomach. However, take it with a small amount of food if the drug is irritating to your stomach. Talk with your doctor, nurse or pharmacist if you feel that the drug is not working effectively.

A-51

Drug: **Antibiotics**

Food: Folic acid, magnesium, potassium, vitamins (e.g., B_6, B_{12}, K)

Outcome: Antibiotics can inactivate or interfere with the normal absorption and activity of these nutrients.

What to Do: Antibiotics are usually taken for less than 2 weeks, so it is unlikely that this interaction will cause problems. Eat a balanced diet. Your doctor will recommend dietary changes if they are indicated.

A-52

Drug: **Anticholinergics**

Food: Food in general

Outcome: Food can interfere with normal absorption of these drugs, which can reduce therapeutic effectiveness.

What to Do: Try to take the drug 1 hour before or 2 hours after eating. Notify your doctor, nurse or pharmacist if you feel that the drug is not working.

A-53

Drug: **Anticoagulants ("blood thinners")**

Food: Alcohol

Outcome: Mixed reports (both increased and decreased drug activity) have appeared in the medical literature.

What to Do: Avoid alcohol while on anticoagulant therapy until you consult a health professional. Notify your doctor of any unusual symptoms, such as bleeding or bruising. Keep all laboratory and clinic appointments in order that your therapy can be effectively monitored.

A-54

Drug: **Anticoagulants ("blood thinners")**

Food: Cooking oils with silicone additives

Outcome: Cooking oils of this type can bind with these drugs to form a nutrient/drug complex that is not absorbed normally.

What to Do: Avoid cooking oils with silicone additives if you are taking anticoagulants.

A-55

Drug: **Anticoagulants ("blood thinners")**

Food: Vitamin B complex

Outcome: Decreased effectiveness of the drug has been reported.

What to Do: Eat a balanced diet. Your doctor will recommend dietary changes if they are indicated. Keep all laboratory and clinic appointments. These are necessary for appropriate monitoring of your therapy.

A-56

Drug: **Anticoagulants ("blood thinners")**

Food: Vitamin C

Outcome: Large doses of the vitamin (3+ grams/day) can interfere with normal absorption of the drug. This can result in decreased effectiveness of therapy.

What to Do: Eat a balanced diet. Avoid excessive intake of the vitamin. Your doctor will recommend dietary changes if they are indicated. Notify your doctor, nurse or pharmacist if your therapy does not seem to be working effectively.

A-57

Drug: **Anticoagulants ("blood thinners")**

Food: Vitamin E

Outcome: Large doses (1,200+U/day) may increase drug activity (including adverse effects) and bleeding risk.

What to Do: Eat a balanced diet. Your doctor will recommend dietary changes if they are indicated. It is best to avoid excessive intake of vitamin supplements without first consulting a health professional. Report any unusual symptoms to your doctor, nurse or pharmacist. Keep all laboratory and clinic appointments. These are necessary to monitor the effectiveness of your therapy.

A-58

Drug: **Anticoagulants ("blood thinners")**

Food: Foods rich in vitamin K (see Appendix 2)

Outcome: Vitamin K can interfere with the ability of the drug to work effectively.

What to Do: Eat a balanced diet. Avoid excessive intake of foods rich in vitamin K. Check with your doctor about special diets or nutritional needs while you are on therapy. Keep all clinic and laboratory appointments. These are necessary for appropriate monitoring of your therapy.

A-59

Drug: **Anticoagulants ("blood thinners")**

Food: Vegetables

Outcome: Excessive intake of some vegetables (see Appendix 2) can interfere with the ability of the drug to work effectively.

What to Do: Eat a balanced diet. Avoid excessive intake of foods rich in vitamin K. Check with your doctor about special diets or nutritional needs while you are on therapy. Keep all clinic and laboratory appointments. These are necessary for appropriate monitoring of your therapy.

A-60

Drug: **Anticonvulsants**

Food: Alcohol

Outcome: Alcohol can interfere with the ability of these drugs to control seizures.

What to Do: Avoid alcoholic beverages while on therapy without first checking with your doctor, nurse or pharmacist.

A-61

Drug: **Anticonvulsants**

Food: Calcium

Outcome: Decreased calcium levels can occur because of effects which these drugs have on metabolic activities in the body.

What to Do: Eat a balanced diet. Your doctor will recommend dietary changes if they are indicated. Report any unusual symptoms (see Appendix 12) to your doctor, nurse or pharmacist.

A-62

Drug: **Anticonvulsants**

Food: Folic acid

Outcome: Vitamin depletion and deficiency have been reported. However, supplementation can interfere with the normal activity of the drug and increase seizure risk.

What to Do: Eat a balanced diet. Keep all medical and laboratory appointments so that your therapy can be monitored carefully. Your doctor will recommend dietary changes or supplements if they are indicated. Report any unusual symptoms (see Appendix 13) to your doctor, nurse or pharmacist.

A-63

Drug: **Anticonvulsants**

Food: Vitamin D

Outcome: The drug can inactivate the vitamin and increase its excretion; vitamin deficiency is possible.

What to Do: Eat a balanced diet. Your doctor will recommend dietary changes if they are indicated. Vitamin supplementation (e.g., 400-800 International Units / day) and a diet rich in calcium are sometimes recommended. Report any unusual symptoms (see Appendix 25) to your doctor, nurse or pharmacist.

A-64

Drug: **Anticonvulsants**

Food: Vitamin K

Outcome: Inactivation of vitamin K can occur.

What to Do: Your doctor will recommend dietary or therapeutic changes if they are indicated. Report any unusual symptoms (see Appendix 27) to your doctor, nurse or pharmacist.

A-65

Drug: **Antidepressants (e.g., Tricyclics)**

Food: Alcohol

Outcome: Excessive (and possibly dangerous) sedation and depression of the central nervous system is possible (e.g., incoordination, impaired judgment, decreased performance skills and alertness, slowed reaction time, dizziness, increased risk of falls). Both alcohol and these drugs can cause dizziness when arising quickly from a seated or lying position. Additionally, alcohol can increase the likelihood of depression.

What to Do: Avoid alcohol with antidepressant therapy without first consulting a health professional. Avoid taking the medication and alcohol within 3-4 hours of each other. Avoid arising too quickly from a seated or lying position.

A-66

Drug: **Antihistamines**

Food: Alcohol

Outcome: Excessive (and possibly dangerous) sedation and depression of the central nervous system is possible (e.g., incoordination, impaired judgment, decreased performance skills and alertness, slowed reaction time, dizziness, increased risk of falls), especially with sedating antihistamines.

What to Do: Avoid alcohol use while on antihistamine therapy without first talking with a health professional.

A-67

Drug: **Antihistamines**

Food: Foods that acidify the urine (see Appendix 4)

Outcome: Antihistamines are excreted more quickly in acid urine. This can result in decreased drug levels and reduced drug activity.

What to Do: This interaction is not likely to occur unless you are taking large amounts of these foods. Notify your doctor, nurse or pharmacist if your therapy does not seem to be working.

A-68

Drug: **Antihistamine**

Food: Foods that produce alkaline urine (see Appendix 5)

Outcome: Antihistamines are not excreted as quickly as normal in alkaline urine. This can result in increased drug levels and activity (e.g., sedation, dryness of the mouth and eyes).

What to Do: This interaction is not likely to occur unless you are taking large amounts of these foods. Notify your doctor, nurse or pharmacist if you experience new or more severe symptoms of any kind.

A-69

Drug: **Antihypertensives**

Food: Alcohol

Outcome: Alcohol dilates blood vessels, which can result in dizziness and fainting, especially when arising from a seated or lying position. The results are unpredictable depending upon the drug involved. Long-term alcohol use can cause your blood pressure to increase.

What to Do: Avoid alcohol if you are taking medications for high blood pressure without first consulting a health professional.

A-70

Drug: **Antihypertensives (Ganglionic Blockers)**

Food: Food in general

Outcome: Food can interfere with normal absorption of the drug.

What to Do: Take the medication 1 hour before or 2 hours after eating. Notify your doctor, nurse or pharmacist if the drug does not seem to be working effectively.

A-71

Drug: **Antihypertensives**

Food: Licorice (natural)

Outcome: Natural licorice counteracts the anti-hypertensive effects of the drug. Blood pressure increases because of sodium and water retention.

What to Do: Since licorice is not a frequent item in most diets, there is probably little cause for concern. Also, most "licorice" products commonly sold in the U.S. contain licorice flavoring instead of natural licorice. Blood pressure should be checked on a regular basis. Notify your doctor if the drug seems not to be working.

A-72

Drug: **Antihypertensives**

Food: Sodium (salt)

Outcome: Salt causes water retention. This means that more fluid is being pumped in the blood vessels, so blood pressure increases.

What to Do: The average American diet has 10 times the amount of salt actually needed by the body for normal functioning. So, cutting back would probably be healthier for everyone, but especially if you have high blood pressure. An easy way for most people to reduce their salt intake is to use it only at the table, but not in cooking. Also, lemon can be used as a salt substitute on appropriate foods. Your doctor may recommend more strict salt diets depending upon the severity of your blood pressure problem. Be aware of foods with a high sodium content (see Appendix 1).

A-73

Drug: **Anti-Inflammatory Agents (NSAIDs, phenylbutazone, indomethacin)**

Food: Sodium

Outcome: These drugs and salt can both contribute to the retention of water and an increase in blood pressure.

What to Do: Have regular blood pressure checks if you take these drugs regularly. The risk for a problem is usually low in most people unless health problems exist (e.g., high blood pressure, kidney disease).

A-74

Drug: **Antipsychotics**

Food: Alcohol

Outcome: Excessive (and possibly dangerous) sedation and depression of the central nervous system is possible (e.g., uncoordination, impaired judgment, decreased performance skills and alertness, slowed reaction time, dizziness, increased risk of falls).

What to Do: Avoid this mix.

A-75

Drug: **Antipsychotics**

Food: Coffee, tea

Outcome: Coffee and tea can reduce the effectiveness of these drugs. Also, caffeine is a stimulant, which can cause a problem for some patients being treated for mental health problems.

What to Do: Notify your doctor if your therapy does not seem to be working effectively.

A-76

Drug: **Antipsychotics**

Food: Vitamin B_2

Outcome: Some of these drugs can interfere with the normal metabolism of vitamin B_2; mild deficiencies have been reported.

What to Do: Eat a balanced diet, including foods rich in B vitamins (e.g., milk; cheese; green, leafy vegetables). Report any unusual symptoms (see Appendix 20) to your doctor, nurse or pharmacist.

A-77

Drug: **Antituberculars**

Food: Folic acid, vitamin B_3 (niacin, nicotinic acid), vitamin B_6 (pyridoxine)

Outcome: Vitamin depletion and vitamin deficiencies are possible with long-term use.

What to Do: Eat a balanced diet. Your doctor will prescribe nutritional supplements or dietary changes if they are indicated. Report any unusual symptoms (see Appendices 13, 21, 19, 22, 23) to your doctor, nurse or pharmacist.

A-78

Drug: **Aspirin**

Food: Alcohol

Outcome: Both aspirin and alcohol are irritating to the stomach. When taken together, there is a much greater risk of irritation, ulcers and bleeding of the esophagus and stomach. Also, increased blood alcohol levels have been reported.

What to Do: Avoid this mix.

A-79

Drug: **Aspirin**

Food: Caffeine

Outcome: Caffeine can increase aspirin absorption, which can result in higher drug levels, activity and adverse effects. Also, this combination is more likely to result in irritation of the stomach.

What to Do: It is probably best to avoid taking aspirin with caffeine-containing beverages. It is best to take aspirin with a full glass of water.

A-80

Drug: **Aspirin**

Food: Food in general

Outcome: It is thought that food can decrease aspirin absorption.

What to Do: Aspirin is usually taken with food to reduce stomach irritation.

A-81

Drug: **Aspirin**

Food: Folic acid

Outcome: Folic acid deficiency is possible. Folic acid is carried throughout the body on special carrier molecules. Aspirin competes with folic acid for this carrier, so that less folic acid reaches the tissues that need it. "Pseudosenility" has been reported in elderly.

What to Do: Eat a balanced diet. Folic acid supplementation is not usually necessary, even for people on long-term aspirin therapy (e.g., for arthritis). Report any unusual symptoms (see Appendix 13) to your doctor, nurse or pharmacist.

A-82

Drug: **Aspirin**

Food: Foods that acidify the urine (see Appendix 4)

Outcome: Aspirin is not excreted normally in acid urine. This would allow aspirin levels, activity and adverse effects to increase.

What to Do: Eat a balanced diet. This interaction should not be a problem unless large amounts of these foods are being consumed. Report any unusual symptoms (e.g., stomach irritation; heartburn; ringing in the ears; black, tar-like stools; "coffee grounds" vomit) to your doctor, nurse or pharmacist.

A-83

Drug: **Aspirin**

Food: Herbal teas (e.g., sweet clover, woodruff, tonka bean)

Outcome: These teas contain natural sources of coumarin (a "blood thinner"). Aspirin also thins the blood. This interaction can interfere with the ability of the blood to clot normally and increase the risk of bleeding.

What to Do: Reduce intake or avoid these teas while on therapy.

A-84

Drug: **Aspirin**

Food: Iron

Outcome: Both iron and aspirin are irritating to the stomach. Iron-deficiency anemia has been reported, possibly due to bleeding of the stomach or intestines.

What to Do: It is best to take iron and aspirin with food in order to reduce the risk of stomach distress and bleeding. Anemia has only been reported with long-term use. Discuss any supplementation concerns with your doctor, nurse or pharmacist.

A-85

Drug: **Aspirin (enteric-coated)**

Food: Milk, alkaline foods

Outcome: Enteric coatings dissolve in the alkaline environment of the intestines, rather than the acid environment of the stomach. This reduces the risk of stomach irritation by aspirin. Alkaline foods may cause this protective enteric-coating to dissolve prematurely.

What to Do: It is always best to take aspirin products with a full glass of water. Water facilitates absorption, reduces the risk of irritation to the stomach and intestines, and will not cause the protective enteric coating to dissolve prematurely.

A-86

Drug: **Aspirin**

Food: Potassium

Outcome: Potassium depletion has been reported with large doses of aspirin.

What to Do: It is unlikely that this problem would occur unless large doses of aspirin are being taken for long time periods. Report any unusual symptoms (see Appendix 16) to your doctor, nurse or pharmacist.

A-87

Drug: **Aspirin**

Food: Sugar

Outcome: Excessive sugar intake combined with large doses of aspirin has been reported to decrease sexual activity.

What to Do: Eat a balanced diet. Avoid excessive intake of sugar for general health.

A-88

Drug: **Aspirin**

Food: Vitamin C (ascorbic acid)

Outcome: Aspirin can increase the excretion of vitamin C, which can result in decreased vitamin C levels.

What to Do: Vitamin deficiencies are unlikely, since vitamins are consumed daily in food. Report any unusual symptoms (see Apendix 24) to your doctor, nurse or pharmacist.

A-89

Drug: **Astemizole**

Food: Food in general

Outcome: Food can interfere with normal absorption of astemizole.

What to Do: It is best to take the drug on an empty stomach (i.e., 1 hour before or 2 hours after meals).

A-90

Drug: **Atabrine**

Food: Alcohol

Outcome: Atabrine interferes with normal alcohol metabolism, which can result in a disulfiram-like reaction (see Appendix 11).

What to Do: Avoid alcohol while taking this drug.

A-91

Drug: **Atenolol**

Food: Alcohol

Outcome: Contradictory reports exist regarding the effects of alcohol on beta-blockers. Unpredictable effects may occur depending upon the condition being treated.

What to Do: In general, alcohol should be avoided by anyone being treated for blood pressure or heart problems, since long-term use can increase blood pressure and damage heart muscle.

A-92

Drug: **Atenolol**

Food: Calcium

Outcome: Decreased drug activity has been reported.

What to Do: Eat a balanced diet. Your doctor will recommend dietary changes if they are indicated. It is best to avoid supplementation (especially excessive amounts) without first consulting with a health professional. Notify your doctor, nurse or pharmacist if your therapy does not seem to be working effectively.

A-93

Drug: **Atenolol**

Food: Food in general

Outcome: Food can interfere with the absorption of many drugs.

What to Do: Report any unusual symptoms or lack of effectiveness to your doctor, nurse or pharmacist.

A-94

Drug: **Atovaquone**

Food: Food in general

Outcome: Food enhances absorption of the drug, resulting in higher blood levels.

What to Do: It is recommended that the drug *should* be taken with food.

A-95

Drug: **Atropine**

Food: Foods that acidify the urine (see Appendix 4)

Outcome: Atropine is excreted more quickly than normal in acid urine. This can result in decreased drug activity.

What to Do: Eat a balanced diet. Avoid excessive intake of these foods. Your doctor will recommend dietary changes of they are indicated. Notify your doctor, nurse or pharmacist if your therapy does not seem to be working effectively.

A-96

Drug: **Azithromycin**

Food: Food in general

Outcome: Food can decrease absorption and effects of azithromycin.

What to Do: Take on an empty stomach (1 hour before or 2 hours after eating).

A-97

Drug: **Azulfidine**

Food: Folic acid

Outcome: The drug can block normal uptake of folic acid by the body, resulting in a deficiency.

What to Do: Eat a balanced diet. Your doctor will recommend nutritional supplementation if it is indicated. Report any unusual symptoms (see Appendix 13) to your doctor, nurse or pharmacist.

B-1

Drug: **Baking Soda (antacid)**

Food: Sodium (salt)

Outcome: Mixing baking soda (sodium bicarbonate) and salt (sodium chloride) can result in increased sodium levels (see Appendix 17). This can result in fluid retention, increased blood pressure and decreased effectiveness of medications used to treat high blood pressure.

What to Do: The average American diet has 10 times the amount of salt actually needed by the body for normal functioning. So, cutting back would probably be healthier for everyone, but especially if you have high blood pressure. An easy way for most people to reduce their salt intake is to use it sparingly at the table, but not in cooking. Also, lemon can be used as a salt substitute on appropriate foods. Your doctor may recommend more strict salt diets if your blood pressure is a problem. Sodium bicarbonate is not usually the best choice when antacids are needed. Ask your doctor, nurse or pharmacist to recommend an appropriate antacid for your needs.

B-2

Drug: **Barbiturates**

Food: Alcohol

Outcome: Excessive (and possibly dangerous) sedation and depression of the central nervous system is possible (e.g., uncoordination, impaired judgment, decreased performance skills and alertness, slowed reaction time, dizziness, increased risk of falls). Short-term use of alcohol can interfere with the normal metabolism, which can result in increased blood levels, activity and adverse effects of barbiturates. Chronic alcohol ingestion can cause the liver to metabolize the drug more quickly. In this case, lower blood levels and activity of the drug may occur.

What to Do: Avoid this mix.

B-3

Drug: **Barbiturates**

Food: Charcoal-broiled food

Outcome: These foods may cause barbiturates to be metabolized by the body more quickly than normal. This could reduce the effectiveness of the drug.

What to Do: This outcome is unlikely unless large or consistent amounts of these foods are being consumed. Contact your doctor, nurse or pharmacist if your drug therapy does not seem to be working effectively.

B-4

Drug: **Barbiturates**

Food: Folic acid

Outcome: Decreased folic acid levels and deficiencies are possible.

What to Do: Eat a balanced diet. Your doctor will recommend dietary changes or supplements if they are indicated. Report any unusual symptoms (see Appendix 13) to your doctor, nurse or pharmacist.

B-5

Drug: **Barbiturates**

Food: Foods that acidify the urine (see Appendix 4)

Outcome: Barbiturates are not excreted normally in acid urine. Increased drug levels, activity and adverse effects of the drug are possible.

What to Do: Problems are unlikely unless large amounts of these foods are being consumed. Eat a balanced diet. Notify your doctor, nurse or pharmacist if you begin to experience more pronounced side effects (e.g., sedation, loss of coordination).

B-6

Drug: **Barbiturates**

Food: Foods that produce alkalinize urine (see Appendix 5)

Outcome: Barbiturates are more rapidly excreted in alkaline urine. This results in lower levels and activity of the drug.

What to Do: Eat a balanced diet. This interaction is unlikely unless large amounts of these foods are being consumed. Notify your doctor, nurse or pharmacist if your therapy does not seem to be working effectively.

B-7

Drug: **Barbiturates**

Food: Protein-deficient diets

Outcome: Barbiturates are not metabolized normally if a protein-deficient diet is being consumed. This can result in increased drug levels, activity and adverse effects of these drugs.

What to Do: Eat a balanced diet. Notify your doctor, nurse or pharmacist if you begin to experience more pronounced side effects (e.g., sedation, uncoordination).

B-8

Drug: **Barbiturates**

Food: Sugars (glucose, fructose, sucrose)

Outcome: Research in laboratory animals indicates that sugars may interfere with the normal metabolism of barbiturates. This could result in increased activity and adverse effects.

What to Do: Animal studies are not always accurate predictors of drug activity in humans. Even if this problem can occur, it would likely only occur if large amounts of sugars are being consumed. Notify your doctor, nurse or pharmacist if you begin to experience more pronounced side effects (e.g., sedation, incoordination).

B-9

Drug: **Barbiturates**

Food: Vitamin B_{12}, vitamin D

Outcome: Barbiturates can result in an increased need for these vitamins.

What to Do: Eat a balanced diet. Supplementation should not be necessary with short-term drug therapy. Your doctor will recommend dietary changes if they are indicated. Notify your doctor, nurse or pharmacist if you experience unusual symptoms (see Appendices 23 and 25).

B-10

Drug: **Benzodiazepines**

Food: Alcohol

Outcome: Excessive (and possibly dangerous) sedation and depression of the central nervous system is possible (e.g., uncoordination, impaired judgment, decreased performance skills and alertness, slowed reaction time, dizziness, increased risk of falls).

What to Do: Avoid this mix.

B-11

Drug: **Benzodiazepines**

Food: Caffeine, coffee, tea, cola beverages

Outcome: Caffeine can interfere with the normal activity of benzodiazepines. The clinical impact of this interaction is not well understood.

What to Do: It is best to avoid caffeine (especially excessive intake) to achieve the most effective therapy. Notify your doctor, nurse or pharmacist if the drug does not seem to be working effectively. Always exercise caution when driving or engaging in activities that require mental alertness after taking benzodiazepines.

Caffeine could cause you to feel more alert than you really are.

B-12

Drug: **Benzodiazepines**

Food: Charcoal-broiled foods

Outcome: These foods can increase metabolism of benzodiazepines. This could cause the drug to be eliminated more quickly than normal.

What to Do: Avoid excessive intake of these foods while on therapy. Notify your doctor, nurse or pharmacist if the drug does not seem to be working effectively.

B-13

Drug: **Benzodiazepines**

Food: Food in general

Outcome: Food can interfere with the normal absorption of benzodiazepines. Other reports suggest that food may increase the absorption, levels and activity of these drugs.

What to Do: Notify your doctor, nurse or pharmacist if you feel that your therapy is not working effectively, or if you experience unusual symptoms or adverse drug effects while on therapy.

B-14

Drug: **Benzodiazepines**

Food: Smoking

Outcome: Smoking may increase normal metabolism of the drug. This could cause the drug to be eliminated from the body more quickly than normal.

What to Do: Smoking is hazardous to your health in general. So, it is best to quit. Notify your doctor, nurse or pharmacist if your therapy does not seem to be working.

B-15

Drug: **Beta-Blockers**

Food: Alcohol

Outcome: Contradictory reports exist on the effects of alcohol on beta-blockers. Unpredictable effects have been reported depending upon the drug involved and the condition being treated.

What to Do: It is best to avoid this mix.

B-16

Drug: **Beta-Blockers**

Food: Calcium

Outcome: Decreased blood levels and activity of some beta-blockers are possible.

What to Do: Eat a balanced diet. Your doctor will recommend

dietary changes if they are indicated. It is probably best to avoid excessive intake of calcium (e.g., supplementation) without first consulting with a health professional. Notify your doctor, nurse or pharmacist if your therapy does not seem to be working effectively or if any unusual symptoms occur.

B-17

Drug: **Biguanides**

Food: Glucose

Outcome: Biguanides can interfere with the normal absorption of glucose.

What to Do: No interventions are necessary. The average American diet usually has an ample supply of sugars.

B-18

Drug: **Biguanides**

Food: Vitamin B_{12}

Outcome: Vitamin depletion and anemia have been reported.

What to Do: Eat a balanced diet. Vitamin levels are normally maintained by the diet. Your doctor will recommend dietary changes or supplements if they are indicated. Notify your doctor, nurse or pharmacist if unusual symptoms occur (see Appendix 23).

B-19

Drug: **Bile Acid Sequestrants**

Food: Beta carotene, vitamins A, B_{12}, D, E, K, iron, lipids

Outcome: Decreased absorption of these nutrients can occur.

What to Do: Eat a balanced diet. Ample vitamin intake is normally supplied in the diet. Notify your doctor, nurse or pharmacist if unusual symptoms appear (see Appendices 18, 23, 25, 26, 27).

B-20

Drug: **Bisacodyl**

Food: Alkaline foods (e.g., milk, dairy products, vegetables, almonds, chestnuts)

Outcome: The foods can cause the enteric coating on this drug to dissolve in the stomach instead of the intestines. When bisacodyl is released in the stomach it can cause significant stomach irritation and abdominal cramping.

What to Do: Take this drug on an empty stomach (1 hour before or 2 hours after meals). It is best to take it with water, rather than other beverages.

B-21

Drug: **Bisacodyl**

Food: Calcium, fat, food in general, glucose, potassium

Outcome: Bisacodyl can interfere with the normal absorption or excretion of these nutrients.

What to Do: Eat a healthy diet. Notify your doctor, nurse or pharmacist if you experience any unusual symptoms (see Appendices 12, 16). Never use laxatives for more than a week without first consulting a health professional.

B-22

Drug: **Blood Pressure Medications**

Food: Alcohol

Outcome: Alcohol can have unpredictable effects on blood pressure therapy. Alcohol dilates blood vessels, which can result in drops in blood pressure, dizziness and fainting, especially when arising from a seated or lying position. Also, alcohol can mask pain that normally serves as a warning signal of problems. Long-term alcohol use can damage heart muscles.

What to Do: It is best to avoid alcohol while on therapy.

B-23

Drug: **Brompheniramine**

Food: Alcohol

Outcome: Excessive (and possibly dangerous) sedation and depression of the central nervous system is possible (e.g., uncoordination, impaired judgment, decreased performance skills and alertness, slowed reaction time, dizziness, increased risk of falls).

What to Do: Avoid this mix.

B-24

Drug: **Bronchodilators**

Food: Caffeine, coffee, tea

Outcome: Both caffeine and bronchodilators have stimulant effects. When taken together, increased side effects may occur.

What to Do: Consider reducing your intake of caffeinated beverages while on therapy.

B-25

Drug: **Bronchodilators**

Food: High-protein, low-carbohydrate diets

Outcome: These foods could theoretically increase metabolism of the drug. This would reduce drug levels and activity.

What to Do: This type of diet can be hazardous to your health. Interference with bronchodilator therapy can be dangerous when it is truly needed.

B-26

Drug: **Buspirone**

Food: Alcohol

Outcome: In normal therapeutic ranges, the drug does *not* appear to potentiate the sedative and depressant effects of alcohol.

What to Do: It is best to avoid alcohol use with all drug therapy.

B-27

Drug: **Buspirone**

Food: Food in general

Outcome: Food can reduce absorption, but also appears to decrease metabolism. So, the overall effect is unlikely to be significant.

What to Do: No interventions are indicated.

C-1

Drug: **Caffeine**

Food: Grapefruit juice

Outcome: Increased drug levels, duration of action and activity (including adverse drug effects) of caffeine can occur.

What to Do: Be aware that this combination may result in a greater likelihood of adverse caffeine effects than normal (e.g., nervousness, increased heart rate, a pounding sensation in the chest, increased blood pressure).

C-2

Drug: **Caffeine**

Food: Smoking

Outcome: Smoking increases elimination of caffeine.

What to Do: The elimination of caffeine is not considered to be a problem. Smoking is hazardous to health in general. It is best to quit.

C-3

Drug: **Calcium**

Food: Chocolate, oxalic acid (e.g., spinach), phytic acid (e.g., nuts, legumes and cereal grains).

Outcome: These foods can bind with calcium, reducing its normal absorption.

What to Do: This interaction is ulikely to cause problems unless large amounts of these foods are being consumed. Eat a balanced diet. Report unusual symptoms (see Appendix 12) to your doctor, nurse or pharmacist.

C-4

Drug: **Calcium**

Food: Diets high in dietary fiber.

Outcome: Fiber can bind with calcium and interfere with normal absorption of calcium.

What to Do: Eat a balanced diet. Report any unusual symptoms (see Appendix 12) to your doctor, nurse or pharmacist.

C-5

Drug: **Calcium Acetate**

Food: Food in general

Outcome: Calcium acetate binds with phosphates in foods and reduces the amount absorbed from the diet.

What to Do: This drug is used to decrease phosphate levels in patients with kidney disease. Take the drug with meals as directed.

C-6

Drug: **Calcium Carbimide (citrated)**

Food: Alcohol

Outcome: This drug can interfere with the normal metabolism of alcohol, resulting in a disulfiram-like reaction (see Appendix 11).

What to Do: Avoid this mix.

C-7

Drug: **Calcium Carbonate**

Food: Fats

Outcome: Fat and calcium are bound together in the gut, so that higher than normal levels of fats are lost in the stool. It is worth noting that excessive fat intake is associated with the development of some cancers. Milk and some calcium products have been reported to reduce the incidence of colon and rectal cancers. Even so, calcium is NOT an antidote for cancers due to poor lifestyle choices (e.g., diets high in fats).

What to Do: No interventions are necessary. Fat lost in this way is not usually a health problem. It is important to eat a balanced diet (no-fat diets can also be unhealthy). Report any unusual symptoms to your doctor.

C-8

Drug: **Calcium Channel Blockers**
[amlodipine, felodipine, nifedipine, nimodipine]

Food: Grapefruit juice

Outcome: Increased absorption, drug levels and activity (including adverse drug effects) of calcium channel blockers can occur.

What to Do: It is best to take medications with water, rather than other fluids. Report any unusual side effects (e.g., flushing, headache, rapid pulse, hypotension) to your doctor, nurse or pharmacist.

C-9

Drug: **Captopril**

Food: Food in general

Outcome: Food can interfere with the absorption of captopril.

What to Do: It is best to take the drug 1 hour before or 2 hours after eating. If stomach distress occurs, talk with your doctor about alternatives.

C-10

Drug: **Carbamazepine**

Food: Food in general

Outcome: Food results in an increase in the production and release of digestive secretions (e.g., enzymes, bile), which causes the drug to dissolve and be absorbed more quickly.

What to Do: This medication is usually taken with food in order to maximize therapy. Report any unusual, disturbing or intolerable side effects to your doctor, nurse or pharmacist.

C-11

Drug: **Carbamazepine**

Food: Vitamin D

Outcome: Vitamin losses and deficiency symptoms have been reported in some patients.

What to Do: Eat a balanced diet. Your doctor will recommend dietary supplements if indicated. Report any unusual symptoms (see Appendix 25) to your doctor, nurse or pharmacist.

C-12

Drug: **Cardiac Glycosides**

Food: Calcium, calcium-containing foods (e.g., milk)

Outcome: Calcium can affect the normal functioning of heart muscle. Excessive calcium levels can increase the risk of toxicity from these drugs (e.g., arrhythmias). Insufficient intake of calcium can decrease the effectiveness of therapy with these drugs.

What to Do: Eat a balanced diet. Your doctor will recommend dietary supplements or changes if they are indicated. Report any unusual symptoms (e.g., unusually slow or irregular pulse) to your doctor, nurse or pharmacist.

C-13

Drug: **Cardiac Glycosides**

Food: Licorice (natural)

Outcome: Natural licorice can lower potassium levels, which in turn, can increase the risk for adverse effects due to these drugs. Natural licorice can also result in sodium and fluid retention, which would tend to increase blood pressure and work load on the heart.

What to Do: Avoid natural licorice when taking these drugs. Most contemporary candies and foods utilize artificial licorice flavoring, which is not a problem for therapy. However, natural licorice can be purchased from health and natural food stores. Always read product labels to see whether commercial products contain natural licorice or artificial flavoring. Report any unusual symptoms (see Appendix 16) to your doctor, nurse or pharmacist.

C-14

Drug: **Cardiac Glycosides**

Food: Magnesium

Outcome: Low magnesium levels can result in an increase in adverse drug effects with this therapy.

What to Do: Eat a balanced diet. Your doctor will recommend dietary supplements or changes if they are indicated. Report any unusual symptoms (see Appendix 15) to your doctor, nurse or pharmacist.

C-15

Drug: **Cardiac Glycosides**

Food: Prune juice, bran cereals, dietary fiber

Outcome: These foods can interfere with the normal absorption of these drugs. This results in decreased drug levels and activity.

What to Do: Try to take these drugs 1 hour before or 2 hours after eating these foods.

C-16

Drug: **Cardiac Glycosides**

Food: Vitamin B_1 (thiamine)

Outcome: Vitamin depletion can occur.

What to Do: Eat a balanced diet. Your doctor will recommend dietary supplements or changes if they are indicated. Report any unusual symptoms (see Appendix 19) to your doctor, nurse or pharmacist.

C-17

Drug: **Cathartics**

Food: Vitamins, minerals (e.g., calcium), electrolytes (e.g., potassium)

Outcome: Laxatives can cause nutrients to be excreted too quickly to be absorbed normally from the stomach and intestines. Nutrient deficiencies are possible with chronic use of laxatives.

What to Do: The short-term use of laxatives does not usually pose nutritional deficiency problems. Avoid chronic laxative use unless prescribed by a health professional. Report any unusual symptoms to your doctor, nurse or pharmacist.

C-18

Drug: **Cefaclor**

Food: Food in general

Outcome: Food can interfere with normal absorption of cefaclor.

What to Do: It is usually best to take antibiotics on an empty stomach (e.g., 1 hour before or 2 hours after eating). However, antibiotics are often taken with food if they are irritating to the stomach or intestines. Talk with your doctor, nurse or pharmacist if you have questions about taking this drug with food.

C-19

Drug: **Cefamandol, Cefoperazone, Cefotetan**

Food: Alcohol

Outcome: Alcohol and many antibiotics are irritating to the stomach. Taking alcohol and antibiotics together can result in significant abdominal distress. Also, an alcohol intolerance reaction (disulfiram-type; see Appendix 11) has been reported. These drugs can apparently interfere with the normal metabolism of alcohol. The reaction can begin 30 minutes after alcohol ingestion and subsides within several hours. The reaction can occur up to 3 days after the last dose of the antibiotic is taken.

What to Do: Avoid this mix. Do not drink during, or for 72 hours after, therapy.

C-20

Drug: **Cefuroxime**

Food: Food in general

Outcome: Food can increase the levels and activity of cefuroxime.

What to Do: It is usually best to take antibiotics on an empty stomach (e.g., 1 hour before or 2 hours after eating). However, antibiotics are often taken with food if they are irritating to the stomach or intestines. Talk with your doctor, nurse or pharmacist if you have questions about taking these drugs with food.

C-21

Drug: **Central Nervous System Depressants**

Food: Caffeine, coffee, tea, cola drinks

Outcome: Caffeine can offset some of the depressant effects of these drugs.

What to Do: This is not necessarily a bad interaction. However, it is best to avoid excessive caffeine intake for general health reasons. Notify your doctor, nurse or pharmacist if your therapy does not seem to be working effectively.

C-22

Drug: **Cephalosporins, Cefamandole, Cefoperazone, Cefotetan, Moxalactam**

Food: Vitamin K

Outcome: Antibiotics can interfere with intestinal bacteria which are normally responsible for the synthesis of vitamin K. This can result in abnormally low levels of vitamin K, interference with normal blood clotting and can result in bleeding disorders.

What to Do: Antibiotic therapy is usually prescribed for 2 weeks or less, so that this problem is unlikely to occur. Eat a balanced diet. Your doctor will recommend dietary supplements or changes if they are indicated. Report any unusual symptoms (see Appendix 27) to your doctor, nurse or pharmacist.

C-23

Drug: **Cephalosporins (oral), Cephalexin, Cephradine**

Food: Food in general

Outcome: Food can interfere with the normal absorption of many antibiotics.

What to Do: It is usually best to take antibiotics on an empty stomach (e.g., 1 hour before or 2 hours after eating). However, antibiotics are often taken with food if they are irritating to the stomach or intestines. Talk with your doctor, nurse or pharmacist if you have questions about taking these drugs with food.

C-24

Drug: **Charcoal (activated)**

Food: Food in general

Outcome: Activated charcoal is sometimes given following drug overdoses (accidental or deliberate). It appears that charcoal is more effective when taken following a meal than on an empty stomach. It has been suggested that the presence of food may slow the absorption of drugs and increase the length of time that the charcoal remains in the stomach (i.e., before it passes into the intestines). Thus, in drug overdoses the presence of food in the stomach may give the charcoal more time to absorb drugs.

What to Do: In cases of drug overdoses it is important to contact a doctor, ambulance, poison information center, hospital or other medical emergency facility for instructions. Follow instructions given to you by emergency medical personnel.

C-25

Drug: **Chloral Hydrate**

Food: Alcohol

Outcome: This mix can result in excessive (and possibly dangerous) sedation and depression of the central nervous system (e.g., loss of coordination, impaired judgment, decreased performance skills and alertness, slowed reaction time, increased risk of falls). A disulfiram-like reaction (e.g., flushing, increased pulse and respiration) has also been reported. With long-term use, each drug can interfere with the normal metabolism of the other.

What to Do: Avoid this mix.

C-26

Drug: **Chloramphenicol**

Food: Alcohol

Outcome: This drug can interfere with the normal metabolism of alcohol, resulting in a disulfiram-type reaction (Appendix 11).

What to Do: Avoid this mix.

C-27

Drug: **Chloramphenicol**

Food: Amino acids, calcium, fats, folic acid, food in general, magnesium, proteins, vitamins (B_6, B_{12})

Outcome: Chloramphenicol can interfere with the absorption, metabolism or utilization of these nutrients.

What to Do: Eat a balanced diet. Your doctor will recommend dietary supplements or changes if they are indicated. Antibiotics are usually taken for less than 2 weeks, so interactions of this type are unlikely to occur. Report any unusual symptoms (see Appendices 12, 13, 15, 22, 23) to your doctor, nurse or pharmacist.

C-28

Drug: **Chloramphenicol**

Food: Iron

Outcome: Chloramphenicol may reduce the effectiveness of iron supplements in patients who are being treated for anemia. Other reports indicate that increased iron levels may occur.

What to Do: Eat a balanced diet. Your doctor will recommend dietary changes or supplements if they are required. Report unusual symptoms (see Appendix 14) to your doctor, nurse or pharmacist.

C-29

Drug: **Chloramphenicol**

Food: Vitamin K

Outcome: Antibiotics can interfere with intestinal bacteria which are normally responsible for the synthesis of vitamin K. This can result in abnormally low levels of vitamin K, interference with normal blood clotting and bleeding disorders.

What to Do: Eat a balanced diet. Your doctor will recommend dietary supplements or changes if they are indicated. Antibiotics are usually taken for less than 2 weeks, so interactions of this type are unlikely to occur. Report any unusual symptoms (see Appendix 27) to your doctor, nurse or pharmacist.

C-30

Drug: **Chlordiazepoxide**

Food: Alcohol

Outcome: This mix can result in excessive (and possibly dangerous) sedation and depression of the central nervous system (e.g., loss of coordination, impaired judgment, decreased performance skills and alertness, slowed reaction time, increased risk of falls).

What to Do: Avoid this mix.

C-31

Drug: **Chlordiazepoxide**

Food: Caffeine, coffee, tea, cola beverages

Outcome: Caffeine can interfere with the normal effects of this drug, although the results are unpredictable.

What to Do: It may be best to reduce caffeine intake while on therapy. Notify your doctor, nurse or pharmacist if your therapy does not seem to be working effectively. Caffeine could cause you to feel more alert than you really are.

C-32

Drug: **Chlorhexidine**

Food: Food in general

Outcome: The drug can alter taste perception. Tooth discoloration can occur if the drug is taken after meals due to an interaction between some foods and the drug.

What to Do: Use this drug only as directed by your dentist or physician. Keep scheduled appointments for reevaluation while on therapy. Report tooth discoloration to your dentist.

C-33

Drug: **Chloroquine**

Food: Foods that acidify the urine (see Appendix 4)

Outcome: Chloroquine is excreted more quickly than normal in acidic urine. This can result in decreased drug levels and therapeutic effects.

What to Do: Eat a balanced diet. This interaction is not likely to occur unless large amounts of these foods are being consumed. Inform your doctor if your therapy does not seem to be working.

C-34

Drug: **Chloroquine**

Food: Foods that produce alkaline urine (see Appendix 5)

Outcome: Chloroquine is not eliminated from the body as quickly in alkaline urine. This could result in increased drug levels and activity (including adverse drug effects).

What to Do: Eat a balanced diet. This interaction is not likely to occur unless large amounts of these foods are consumed. Report any unusual symptoms or adverse drug effects to your doctor, nurse or pharmacist.

C-35

Drug: **Chloroquine**

Food: Quinine (e.g., tonic water)

Outcome: In theory, it is possible that quinine might interfere with the normal activity of the drug. However, the actual significance is unknown. Both can affect the heart, so that adverse effects (e.g., lowered blood pressure) are possible under some circumstances. Since the amount of quinine that occurs in foods is quite small, the risk for this interaction is probably quite low.

What to Do: It is probably best to avoid excessive intake of foods and beverages that contain quinine while on therapy.

C-36

Drug: **Chlorothiazide**

Food: Food in general

Outcome: Food can result in increased absorption of chlorothiazide.

What to Do: This interaction is not likely to impact therapy in a significant way. Report any unusual symptoms or adverse drug reactions to your doctor, nurse or pharmacist.

C-37

Drug: **Chlorothiazide**

Food: Potassium

Outcome: Many diuretics ("water pills") can increase potassium losses from the body.

What to Do: Eat a balanced diet. Your doctor will recommend dietary changes if they are indicated. Report any unusual symptoms (see Appendix 16) to your doctor, nurse or pharmacist.

C-38

Drug: **Chlorpheniramine**

Food: Alcohol

Outcome: This mix can result in excessive (and possibly dangerous) sedation and depression of the central nervous system (e.g., loss of coordination, impaired judgment, decreased performance skills and alertness, slowed reaction time, increased risk of falls).

What to Do: Avoid this mix.

C-39

Drug: **Chlorpromazine**

Food: Alcohol

Outcome: This mix can result in excessive (and possibly dangerous) sedation and depression of the central nervous system (e.g., loss of coordination, impaired judgment, decreased performance skills and alertness, slowed reaction time, increased risk of falls).

What to Do: Avoid this mix.

C-40

Drug: **Chlorpromazine**

Food: Food in general

Outcome: Food can interfere with normal absorption of the drug from the stomach.

What to Do: It is usually best to take medications on an empty stomach (i.e., 1 hour before or 2 hours after eating) unless they are irritating to the stomach. Notify your doctor, nurse or pharmacist if your therapy does not seem to be working effectively.

C-41

Drug: **Chlorpromazine**

Food: Vitamin B_2 (riboflavin)

Outcome: The drug can interfere with the normal levels and activity of the vitamin. An increase in urinary excretion could result in a clinical deficiency of the vitamin despite an adequate dietary intake.

What to Do: Eat a balanced diet. Your doctor will recommend dietary supplements or changes if they are indicated. Report any unusual symptoms (see Appendix 20) to your doctor, nurse or pharmacist.

C-42

Drug: **Chlorpropamide**

Food: Alcohol

Outcome: Alcohol may interfere with the ability of the drug to control blood sugar levels. Both decreased and increased blood sugar levels has been reported. The symptoms of exaggerated drug activity ("insulin reaction") include dizziness, weakness, mental confusion, collapse, coma. It has also been reported that chlorpropamide can interfere with normal alcohol absorption and result in a disulfiram-type reaction (Appendix 11).

What to Do: In general, diabetics should avoid alcohol consumption because its use can have unpredictable effects on blood sugar control.

C-43

Drug: **Chlortetracycline**

Food: Food in general

Outcome: Food can interfere with drug absorption. This could result in decreased drug levels, activity and effectiveness.

What to Do: It is best to take antibiotics on an empty stomach (i.e., 1 hour before or 2 hours after eating). If the drug is irritating to your stomach, talk with your doctor, nurse or pharmacist.

C-44

Drug: **Cholestyramine**

Food: Calcium, carotene, cholesterol, electrolytes, fats, lipids, folic acid, iron, nutrients (in general), sugar, triglycerides, vitamins (e.g., A, B_{12}, D, E, K), xylose

Outcome: Cholestyramine can interfere with the absorption of these nutrients; deficiencies are possible.

What to Do: This medication is usually taken before meals. Your doctor will recommend dietary supplements or changes if they are indicated. Report any unusual symptoms (see Appendices 12, 13, 18, 23, 25, 26, 27) to your doctor, nurse or pharmacist.

C-45

Drug: **Cimetidine**

Food: Caffeine, coffee, tea, cola drinks

Outcome: Cimetidine can interfere with the normal metabolism of caffeine. This can result in an increase in caffeine activity and side effects.

What to Do: Consider reducing your caffeine intake while on therapy. Caffeine can result in stomach irritation, which can interfere with the effectiveness of therapy.

C-46

Drug: **Cimetidine**

Food: Food in general

Outcome: Food can interfere with the normal absorption of cimetidine. However, this can actually be beneficial by helping to maintain drug levels in the blood between meals.

What to Do: No interventions are recommended.

C-47

Drug: **Cimetidine**

Food: Iron

Outcome: Cimetidine and iron bind together, which can interfere with normal iron absorption.

What to Do: Avoid taking these within 1 to 2 hours of each other. Report any unusual symptoms (see Appendix 14) to your doctor, nurse or pharmacist.

C-48

Drug: **Cimetidine**

Food: Smoking

Outcome: Smoking can result in stomach irritation and ulcers, and therefore, interferes with the ability of cimetidine to reduce stomach acid production.

What to Do: It is best to quit smoking in an effort to maximize therapy and reduce the risk of ulcer formation.

C-49

Drug: **Cimetidine**

Food: Tyramine-rich foods (see Appendix 7)

Outcome: Severe headache accompanied by a temporary increase in blood pressure has been reported.

What to Do: Avoid excessive intake of these foods. Report any unusual symptoms to your doctor, nurse or pharmacist.

C-50

Drug: **Cinoxacin**

Food: Food in general

Outcome: Food interferes with some aspects of drug absorption, although apparently it is not clinically significant.

What to Do: Cinoxacin may be taken without regard to meals.

C-51

Drug: **Ciprofloxacin**

Food: Caffeine

Outcome: Ciprofloxacin can interfere with the normal metabolism and elimination of caffeine. This could result in an increase in caffeine side effects in individuals who consume caffeine-containing foods and beverages while taking this drug.

What to Do: Consider reducing your caffeine intake while on therapy with this medication.

C-52

Drug: **Ciprofloxacin**

Food: Minerals (iron, copper, zinc, magnesium, calcium, manganese), dairy products, milk, yogurt

Outcome: Ciprofloxacin can bind with minerals present in food and mineral supplements, which interferes with the normal absorption of both. This could result in nutritional deficiencies if taken together for long time periods. There are mixed reports regarding this interaction. Some indicate no problem. The likelihood of the interaction may depend upon the mineral involved.

What to Do: Eat a balanced diet. Antibiotics are usually taken for less than 2 weeks, so nutritional deficiencies are unlikely. It is usually best to take antibiotics on an empty stomach unless they are irritating to the stomach. Your doctor will recommend dietary supplements or changes if they are indicated. Notify your doctor, nurse or pharmacist if you experience unusual symptoms or if your therapy does not seem to be working.

C-53

Drug: **Cisplatin**

Food: Magnesium, phosphate, potassium

Outcome: Cisplatin can result in decreased levels of these nutrients.

What to Do: Eat a balanced diet. Your doctor will recommend dietary supplements or changes if they are indicated. Report any unusual symptoms (see Appendices 15, 16) to your doctor, nurse or pharmacist.

C-54

Drug: **Clarithromycin**

Food: Food in general

Outcome: Food delays absorption and interferes with normal metabolism of clarithromycin.

What to Do: It is best to take antibiotics on an empty stomach (1 hour before or 2 hours after meals). However, clarithromycin can be taken with food if stomach distress occurs.

C-55

Drug: **Clindamycin**

Food: Food, pectin, Kaolin-pectin mixtures

Outcome: These foods can bind with clindamycin and interfere with its absorption.

What to Do: It is usually best to take antibiotics on an empty stomach (1 hour before or 2 hours after meals) unless they are irritating to the stomach.

C-56

Drug: **Clobazam**

Food: Alcohol

Outcome: This mix can result in excessive (and possibly dangerous) sedation and depression of the central nervous system (e.g., loss of coordination, impaired judgment, decreased performance skills and alertness, slowed reaction time, increased risk of falls). Also, alcohol consumption can interfere with the normal ability of the body to eliminate this drug. This can result in higher than normal blood levels and drug activity, including adverse drug reactions.

What to Do: Avoid this mix.

C-57

Drug: **Clofibrate**

Food: Calcium, carbohydrates, carotene, cholesterol, electrolytes, fat, food (in general), iron, sugar, triglycerides, vitamins (A, B_{12}, D, E, K), xylose

Outcome: Clofibrate interferes with the normal absorption of these nutrients.

What to Do: Clofibrate is usually taken before meals. Eat a balanced diet. Your doctor will recommend dietary supplements or changes if they are indicated. Report any unusual symptoms (see Appendices 12, 18, 23, 25, 26, 27) to your doctor, nurse or pharmacist.

C-58

Drug: **Clomipramine**

Food: Alcohol

Outcome: This mix can result in excessive (and possibly dangerous) sedation and depression of the central nervous system (e.g., loss of coordination, impaired judgment, decreased performance skills and alertness, slowed reaction time, increased risk of falls).

What to Do: Avoid this mix.

C-59

Drug: **Clonidine**

Food: Sodium

Outcome: Sodium (salt) can result in fluid retention, which can increase blood pressure and reduce the effectiveness of blood pressure therapy.

What to Do: The average American consumes 10 times the amount of salt actually needed by the body for normally functioning. So, it is best to reduce salt intake. Lemon can be used as a salt substitute on appropriate foods (it fools the taste buds). Also, you can significantly reduce your salt intake by eliminating salt from cooking and using it sparingly at the table. If you have high blood pressure, talk with your doctor about appropriate dietary and lifestyle changes.

C-60

Drug: **Cloxacillin**

Food: Food in general

Outcome: Food can interfere with the normal absorption of many antibiotics.

What to Do: It is usually best to take antibiotics on an empty stomach (e.g., 1 hour before or 2 hours after eating). However, antibiotics are often taken with food if they are irritating to the stomach or intestines. Talk with your doctor, nurse or pharmacist if you have questions about taking these drugs with food.

C-61

Drug: **Cloxacillin**

Food: Fruit juices, carbonated beverages

Outcome: These acid beverages can inactivate cloxacillin.

What to Do: Take antibiotics with water instead of other beverages.

C-62

Drug: **Cocaine**

Food: Alcohol

Outcome: The stimulant effects of cocaine (e.g., increased risk taking) and the effects of alcohol (e.g., reduced judgment and coordination) combine to increase the risk of highway accidents. Also, chronic alcohol consumption is toxic to the heart, while cocaine increases heart rate. This combination can result in heart damage and death.

What to Do: Avoid this mix.

C-63

Drug: **Codeine**

Food: Alcohol

Outcome: This mix can result in excessive (and possibly dangerous) sedation and depression of the central nervous system (e.g., loss of coordination, impaired judgment, decreased performance skills and alertness, slowed reaction time, increased risk of falls).

What to Do: Avoid this mix.

C-64

Drug: **Colchicine**

Food: Amino acids, carotene, cholesterol, electrolytes, fats, nitrogen, potassium, sodium, sugars, vitamins (e.g., B_{12}, D), xylose

Outcome: This drug can interfere with the normal absorption of these nutrients.

What to Do: Eat a balanced diet. Your doctor will recommend dietary supplements and changes if they are indicated. Report any unusual symptoms to your doctor, nurse or pharmacist.

C-65

Drug: **Colestipol**

Food: Cholesterol, fats, lipids, vitamins (A, D, E, K)

Outcome: Colestipol can interfere with the absorption of these nutrients.

What to Do: Eat a balanced diet. Your doctor will recommend dietary changes or supplements if they are indicated. Report any unusual symptoms (see Appendices 18, 25, 27) to your doctor, nurse or pharmacist.

C-66

Drug: **Contraceptives (oral)**

Food: Caffeine

Outcome: Oral contraceptives can interfere with normal caffeine metabolism. As a result, the body is less able to eliminate caffeine. Increased caffeine levels and activity can occur, including adverse effects.

What to Do: It is best to avoid excessive intake of caffeine. If caffeine side effects occur (e.g., increased heart rate and blood pressure, nervousness, anxiety, pounding sensation in the chest), reduce your caffeine intake.

C-67

Drug: **Contraceptives (oral)**

Food: Folic acid, vitamin B_6

Outcome: Contraceptives may deplete levels of these nutrients and result in deficiencies. Estrogens stimulate many reactions in the body, some of which require certain vitamins.

What to Do: Eat a balanced diet. Your doctor will recommend dietary changes or supplements if they are needed. Report any unusual symptoms (see Appendices 13, 22) to your doctor, nurse or pharmacist.

C-68

Drug: **Contraceptives (oral)**

Food: Vitamin A

Outcome: Contraceptives can result in increased levels of the vitamin.

What to Do: Eat a balanced diet. Your doctor will recommend dietary changes if they are needed. It is probably best to avoid excessive supplementation of this vitamin while on therapy. Report any unusual symptoms (see Appendix 18) to your doctor, nurse or pharmacist.

C-69

Drug: **Contraceptives (oral)**

Food: Vitamin C

Outcome: Increased estrogen level and activity (including adverse drug effects) can occur.

What to Do: Eat a balanced diet. Your doctor will recommend dietary changes if they are needed. It is best to avoid excessive vitamin supplementation while on therapy without first consulting a health professional. Report any unusual symptoms to your doctor, nurse or pharmacist.

C-70

Drug: **Copper**

Food: Iron, manganese

Outcome: Copper can interfere with the normal absorption of these nutrients.

What to Do: Eat a balanced diet. Report any unusual symptoms to your doctor, nurse or pharmacist.

C-71

Drug: **Corticosteroids**

Food: Alcohol

Outcome: Stomach irritation can occur.

What to Do: Avoid consumption of alcoholic beverages while taking medications (prescription or nonprescription) without first talking with a health professional.

C-72

Drug: **Corticosteroids**

Food: Calcium, magnesium, potassium, vitamins (B_6, C, D), zinc

Outcome: Increased loss of these nutrients can occur.

What to Do: Eat an appropriate diet. Discuss supplementation with a health professional if you will be taking the drug for an extended period of time. Report unusual symptoms (see Appendices 12, 15, 16, 22, 24, 25, 28)

C-73

Drug: **Corticosteroids**

Food: Sodium

Outcome: Sodium and fluid retention can occur.

What to Do: The average American consumes 10 times the amount of salt actually needed by the body for normally functioning. So, most people should to reduce their salt intake. Lemon can be used as a salt substitute on appropriate foods (it fools the taste buds). Also, you can significantly reduce your salt intake by eliminating salt from cooking and using it sparingly at the table. Talk with your doctor about appropriate dietary and lifestyle changes.

C-74

Drug: **Cortisol**

Food: Vitamin C (ascorbic acid)

Outcome: Cortisol can increase metabolism and loss of vitamin C; vitamin deficiency can occur.

What to Do: Eat a balanced diet. Your doctor will recommend dietary supplements or changes if they are indicated. Report any unusual symptoms (see Appendix 24) to your doctor, nurse or pharmacist.

C-75

Drug: **Coumarin**

Food: Foods that produce alkaline urine (see Appendix 5)

Outcome: Coumarin is excreted more quickly than usual in alkaline urine. This can result in a decrease in drug levels, activity and therapeutic effectiveness.

What to Do: Eat a balanced diet. This interaction is unlikely unless large amounts of these foods are being consumed. Your doctor will recommend dietary changes if they are indicated. Be sure to keep all scheduled appointments with your doctor or for laboratory assessments.

C-76

Drug: **Coumarins**

Food: Foods that acidify the urine (see Appendix 4)

Outcome: Coumarin is not excreted normally in acid urine. This can result in higher drug levels and increased drug effects (including adverse effects).

What to Do: Eat a balanced diet. This interaction is unlikely unless large amounts of these foods are being consumed. Your doctor will recommend dietary changes if they are indicated. Be sure to keep all scheduled appointments with your doctor or for laboratory assessments. Report any unusual symptoms (e.g., bleeding) to your doctor, nurse or pharmacist.

C-77

Drug: **Coumarins**

Food: Vitamin K; foods rich in vitamin K (see Appendix 2)

Outcome: Vitamin K can interfere with the effectiveness of blood thinners.

What to Do: It is best to avoid large amounts of these foods if you are taking blood thinners. Talk with your doctor about appropriate dietary changes.

C-78

Drug: **Cyclophosphamide**

Food: Vitamin A

Outcome: Vitamin A enhances the antitumor effects of the drug (at least in animal studies).

What to Do: Vitamin A can be toxic in high doses. Avoid excessive intake of vitamin A without first talking with your doctor.

C-79

Drug: **Cycloserine**

Food: Alcohol

Outcome: Alcohol increases the risk of epileptic episodes.

What to Do: Avoid this mix.

C-80

Drug: **Cycloserine**

Food: Calcium, magnesium, vitamin B_{12}

Outcome: Cycloserine can interfere with the absorption of these nutrients.

What to Do: Eat a balanced diet while on therapy. Report any unusual symptoms (see Appendices 12, 15, 23) to your doctor, nurse or pharmacist.

C-81

Drug: **Cycloserine**

Food: Folic acid, vitamin B_6 (pyridoxine)

Outcome: Cycloserine can inactivate or interfere with the normal activity of these nutrients.

What to Do: Eat a balanced diet. Your doctor will recommend dietary changes or supplements if they are indicated. Report any unusual symptoms (see Appendices 13, 22) to your doctor, nurse or pharmacist.

C-82

Drug: **Cycloserine**

Food: Vitamin K

Outcome: Cycloserine interferes with intestinal bacteria which are normally responsible for the synthesis of vitamin K. This can result in abnormally low levels of vitamin K, interference with normal blood clotting and bleeding disorders.

What to Do: Eat a healthy and balanced diet. Your doctor will recommend dietary changes or supplements if they are indicated. Report any unusual symptoms (see Appendix 27) to your doctor, nurse or pharmacist.

C-83

Drug: **Cyclosporine**

Food: Food in general

Outcome: Food increases the absorption of cyclosporine.

What to Do: Take as directed. Food may actually be utilized to decrease the cost of therapy because adequate immunosuppression could possibly be achieved at a lower dose.

C-84

Drug: **Cyclosporine**

Food: Grapefruit juice

Outcome: Increased absorption, drug levels and activity (including adverse drug effects) of cyclosporine can occur.

What to Do: It is best to take medications with water, rather than other fluids. Report any unusual side effects or symptoms to your doctor, nurse or pharmacist.

D-1

Drug: **Dapsone**

Food: Para-aminobenzoic acid (PABA)

Outcome: PABA interferes with the normal activity of dapsone.

What to Do: Eat a balanced diet. Your doctor will recommend dietary changes if they are indicated. It is best to avoid vitamin supplementation without first consulting a health professional. Notify your doctor, nurse or pharmacist if your therapy does not seem to be working effectively.

D-2

Drug: **Demeclocycline**

Food: Food in general

Outcome: Food tends to decrease the absorption of drugs in general. This could reduce the effectiveness of therapy.

What to Do: It is best to take antibiotics on an empty stomach (1 hour before or 2 hours after eating). If stomach irritation occurs, talk with your doctor, nurse or pharmacist about options for reducing discomfort.

D-3

Drug: **Demeclocycline**

Food: Milk, dairy products, aluminum, calcium, iron, magnesium, zinc

Outcome: These nutrients bind with tetracycline antibiotics and form a complex that is not absorbed from the intestines. This reduces therapeutic effectiveness.

What to Do: Take tetracycline antibiotics 1 hour before or 2 hours after consuming these nutrients.

D-4

Drug: **Desipramine**

Food: Foods that acidify the urine (see Appendix 4)

Outcome: Desipramine is excreted more quickly than normal in acid urine, which would result in decreased drug levels and therapeutic effects. However, the clinical significance of this interaction is unclear.

What to Do: Eat a balanced diet. This reaction is unlikely unless large amounts of these foods are being consumed. Notify your doctor if therapy seems not to be working effectively.

D-5

Drug: **Desipramine**

Food: Foods that produce alkaline urine (see Appendix 5)

Outcome: Desipramine is not excreted normally in alkaline urine. This could result in increased drug levels and activity (including adverse drug effects). However, the clinical significance of this interaction is unclear.

What to Do: This reaction is unlikely unless large amounts of these foods are being consumed. Notify your doctor, nurse or pharmacist if unusual symptoms or adverse drug effects occur.

D-6

Drug: **Diazepam**

Food: Alcohol

Outcome: This mix can result in excessive (and possibly dangerous) sedation and depression of the central nervous system (e.g., loss of coordination, impaired judgment, decreased performance skills and alertness, slowed reaction time, increased risk of falls). Accidental deaths are possible.

What to Do: Avoid this mix.

D-7

Drug: **Diazepam**

Food: Foods that acidify the urine (see Appendix 4)

Outcome: Diazepam is excreted more quickly than normal in acid urine. This could result in reduced drug levels and activity.

What to Do: Eat a balanced diet. This interaction is unlikely unless large amounts of these foods are being consumed. Notify your doctor if the drug does not seem to be working as expected.

D-8

Drug: **Diazepam**

Food: Food in general

Outcome: Conflicting reports exist. Food would normally be expected to decrease drug absorption, levels and activity. However, food has also been reported to increase the absorption, levels and activity of diazepam (i.e., by causing the drug to remain in the stomach longer, thereby increasing drug absorption from the stomach).

What to Do: No interventions are indicated. Notify your doctor, nurse or pharmacist if you experience unusual symptoms or adverse drug effects while on therapy, or if therapy does not seem to be effective.

D-9

Drug: **Dicloxacillin**

Food: Food in general

Outcome: Food can interfere with the normal absorption of many antibiotics.

What to Do: It is usually best to take antibiotics on an empty stomach (e.g., 1 hour before or 2 hours after eating). However, antibiotics are often taken with food if they are irritating to the stomach or intestines. Talk with your doctor, nurse or pharmacist if you have questions about taking these drugs with food.

D-10

Drug: **Dicoumarol (also Dicumarol)**

Food: Food in general (especially foods high in fat)

Outcome: Food can increase absorption of dicoumarol.

What to Do: No interventions are indicated. Notify your doctor, nurse or pharmacist if you experience any unusual symptoms (e.g., bleeding) or adverse drug effects. Be sure to keep all appointments for medical checkups and laboratory work.

D-11

Drug: **Didanosine**

Food: Food in general

Outcome: Food interferes with the normal absorption of didanosine.

What to Do: It is best to take this drug on an empty stomach (1 hour before or 2 hours after meals). Notify your doctor, nurse or pharmacist if your therapy does not seem to be working effectively.

D-12

Drug: **Digestive Enzymes**

Food: Iron

Outcome: Pancreatic enzymes can interfere with the effectiveness of iron supplements; the mechanism is not known.

What to Do: Eat a balanced diet. Your doctor will recommend dietary changes if they are indicated. Report unusual symptoms (see Appendix 14) to your doctor, nurse or pharmacist.

D-13

Drug: **Digoxin, Digitalis**

Food: Food in general, bran, carbohydrates, fiber, foods high in pectin (e.g., apples, pears).

Outcome: These nutrients can interfere with the absorption of these drugs.

What to Do: It is best to take this drug on an empty stomach (1 hour before or 2 hours after food). Notify your doctor, nurse or pharmacist if you experience any unusual symptoms, adverse drug effects, or if the drug does not seem to be working effectively.

D-14

Drug: **Digoxin, Digitalis**

Food: Foods high in protein or fat

Outcome: This type of diet may interfere with elimination of these drugs.

What to Do: Eat a balanced diet. This interaction is unlikely unless large amounts of these foods are consumed. Notify your doctor, nurse or pharmacist if you experience any unusual symptoms or adverse drug effects.

D-15

Drug: **Digoxin, Digitalis**

Food: Licorice (natural)

Outcome: Natural licorice can lower potassium levels, which in turn, can enhance the actions of digitalis and result in drug toxicity.

What to Do: Avoid natural licorice (read product labels!). Most commercial products in the U.S. use harmless artificial licorice flavoring instead of natural licorice. However, natural products are available from some retail outlets (e.g., health food stores).

D-16

Drug: **Digoxin, Digitalis**

Food: Magnesium

Outcome: Magnesium elimination is increased, which can result in magnesium deficiency. Magnesium deficiency can increase the risk for digoxin toxicity.

What to Do: Eat a balanced diet. Increase intake of magnesium-rich foods (e.g., nuts; fish; whole-grain breads and cereals; green, leafy vegetables). Report any unusual symptoms (see Appendix 15) to your doctor, nurse or pharmacist. Avoid alcohol, which increases magnesium excretion.

D-17

Drug: **Digoxin, Digitalis**

Food: Potassium

Outcome: Low potassium levels increase the risk for toxicity from these drugs.

What to Do: Eat a balanced diet. Talk with your doctor about maintaining proper potassium levels.

D-18

Drug: **Digoxin, Digitalis**

Food: Vitamin D

Outcome: Vitamin D increases calcium levels (e.g., through increased calcium absorption and alterations on the deposit and release of calcium by bone). Calcium affects muscle contraction, including heart muscle. As calcium levels increase, the effects of this drug, including toxicity (e.g., arrhythmias), may increase.

What to Do: Eat a balanced diet. Avoid excessive intake of vitamin D unless instructed otherwise by a health professional. The Recommended Daily Allowance (RDA) for vitamin D is 400 International Units. Read product labels carefully, since many calcium and mineral products also contain vitamin D to increase calcium levels in the body. Periodic exposure to sunlight also helps to satisfy the vitamin D requirements of the body.

D-19

Drug: **Diphenhydramine**

Food: Alcohol

Outcome: This mix can result in excessive (and possibly dangerous) sedation and depression of the central nervous system (e.g., loss of coordination, impaired judgment, decreased performance skills and alertness, slowed reaction time, increased risk of falls).

What to Do: Avoid this mix.

D-20

Drug: **Dirithromycin**

Food: Food in general

Outcome: Food can slow dirithromycin absorption, but overall absorption and the peak blood levels eventually achieved may be increased. However, the clinical impact of these effects is not thought to be significant.

What to Do: The drug may be taken without regard to meals.

D-21

Drug: **Dirithromycin**

Food: Milk, dairy products, calcium

Outcome: Enteric-coated products are designed to dissolve in the intestines rather than the stomach in order to avoid stomach distress. These foods can cause the drug to be released in the stomach.

What to Do: Take with water.

D-22

Drug: **Disopyramide**

Food: Alcohol

Outcome: Alcohol may interfere with normal metabolism of disopyramide. This could reduce elimination and increase levels and activity of the drug in the body.

What to Do: It is always best to avoid mixing alcohol with any drug. However, the actual risk of this interaction is considered to be low. Problems are more likely to occur with excessive or long-term use of alcohol. Report any unusual symptoms or side effects to your doctor, nurse or pharmacist.

D-23

Drug: **Disulfiram**

Food: Alcohol

Outcome: Disulfiram interferes with the normal metabolism of alcohol. This can result in an extremely uncomfortable and potentially dangerous reaction, which has come to be known as the "disulfiram reaction" (see Appendix 11).

What to Do: Avoid this mix. Even small amounts of alcohol can cause serious problems when consumed while taking this drug. Read product labels carefully, since many liquid nonprescription products contain alcohol.

D-24

Drug: **Disulfiram**

Food: Aspartame

Outcome: A disulfiram-type reaction has been reported.

What to Do: It is probably best to avoid aspartame products while taking disulfiram. Report any unusual symptoms (see Appendix 11) to your doctor, nurse or pharmacist.

D-25

Drug: **Disulfiram**

Food: Caffeine

Outcome: Disulfiram interferes with the metabolism of caffeine, so that it is more difficult to eliminate. Increased caffeine levels and activity can occur, including adverse drug effects.

What to Do: It is best to limit caffeine intake while on therapy.

D-26

Drug: **Diuretics**

Food: Calcium, chloride, magnesium, potassium, sodium, vitamin A, zinc

Outcome: Increased excretion of these nutrients can occur with some diuretics, which could result in decreased nutrient levels.

What to Do: Eat a balanced diet. Your doctor will recommend dietary changes and supplements if they are indicated. Discuss nonprescription supplementation of these nutrients with your doctor, nurse or pharmacist. Report any unusual symptoms (Appendices 12, 15-18, 28) to your doctor, nurse or pharmacist.

D-27

Drug: **Diuretics**

Food: Electrolytes (e.g., potassium and sodium, especially with high intake)

Outcome: Electrolytes can interfere with the therapeutic effectiveness of diuretics.

What to Do: Eat a balanced diet. Your doctor will recommend dietary changes and supplements if they are indicated. Avoid fad diets or excessive intake of specific nutrients without first talking with your doctor, nurse or pharmacist.

D-28

Drug: **Diuretics (esp. potassium-depleting)**

Food: Licorice (natural)

Outcome: Natural licorice can cause salt and water retention and result in decreased potassium levels.

What to Do: Avoid natural licorice when taking these drugs. Most licorice used in candies and food preparation is artificial licorice flavoring and not natural licorice. However, natural licorice can be purchased from health and natural food stores. Always read product labels to see whether commercial products contain natural licorice or artificial flavoring. Report unusual symptoms to your doctor, nurse or pharmacist.

D-29

Drug: **Diuretics**

Food: Liver, meat, urates

Outcome: It has been reported that this combination could precipitate gout attacks in susceptible individuals.

What to Do: Problems are unlikely unless large quantities of these foods are being consumed. Discuss appropriate dietary changes with your doctor. Report any unusual symptoms or signs of worsening gout to your physician.

D-30

Drug: **Diuretics**

Food: MSG (monosodium glutamate)

Outcome: The adverse effects of MSG can be intensified by diuretics, especially with long-term use (e.g., chest pain, a tightening sensation of the chest, flushing of the face, headache, facial pressure).

What to Do: No particular interventions are indicated, since it is usually difficult to know which foods contain MSG. Report any unusual symptoms (e.g., those listed above) to your doctor, nurse or pharmacist.

D-31

Drug: **Diuretics**

Food: Potassium, salt substitutes

Outcome: Increased potassium levels can occur with potassium-sparing diuretics. Decreased potassium levels can occur with other diuretics.

What to Do: Eat a balanced diet. Avoid excessive intake of potassium-rich foods if you are taking potassium-sparing diuretics. Your doctor will recommend appropriate dietary changes. Report any unusual symptoms (see Appendix 16) to your doctor, nurse or pharmacist.

D-32

Drug: **Diuretics**

Food: Vitamin B_1

Outcome: Diuretics can cause the vitamin to be excreted more quickly than normal in the urine; deficiency is possible.

What to Do: Eat a balanced diet. Your doctor will recommend dietary changes if they are indicated. Report any unusual symptoms (see Appendix 19) to your doctor, nurse or pharmacist.

D-33

Drug: **Doxorubicin**

Food: Riboflavin (vitamin B_2)

Outcome: The drug can interfere with the metabolism of the vitamin, its normal activity in the body and increase its urinary excretion. This interaction could result in a vitamin deficiency despite an adequate dietary intake.

What to Do: Your doctor will recommend dietary changes or supplements if they are indicated. Report any unusual symptoms (see Appendix 20) to your doctor, nurse or pharmacist.

D-34

Drug: **Doxycycline**

Food: Alcohol

Outcome: Alcohol can affect the normal metabolism and activity of drugs and therapy. Short-term use of alcohol can increase the length of doxycycline activity in the body, while long-term alcohol consumption can decrease its activity.

What to Do: Avoid alcohol consumption while taking drugs without first consulting a health professional. Long-term, excessive consumption of alcohol is a health hazard.

D-35

Drug: **Doxycycline**

Food: Food in general

Outcome: Food can decrease the absorption of most antibiotics, although this problem is apparently not as great with doxycycline as with other tetracyclines.

What to Do: It is best to take antibiotics on an empty stomach (i.e., 1 hour before or 2 hours after food). If stomach distress occurs, talk with your doctor, nurse or pharmacist about alternatives for reducing discomfort.

D-36

Drug: **Doxycycline**

Food: Antacids, dairy products (e.g., milk), calcium, iron, magnesium, zinc

Outcome: Tetracyclines can bind with certain nutrients and form complexes that are not easily absorbed from the intestinal tract. This can result in decreased absorption of the drug and decreased drug effects.

What to Do: It is best to take antibiotics on an empty stomach (i.e., 1 hour before or 2 hours after food). If stomach distress occurs, talk with your doctor, nurse or pharmacist about alternatives for reducing discomfort.

D-37

Drug: **Dronabinol**

Food: Alcohol

Outcome: This mix can result in excessive (and possibly dangerous) sedation and depression of the central nervous system (e.g., loss of coordination, impaired judgment, decreased performance skills and alertness, slowed reaction time, increased risk of falls).

What to Do: Avoid this mix.

D-38

Drug: **DSS (dioctyl sodium sulfosuccinate) and other Surfactants**

Food: Vitamin A

Outcome: Increased absorption of vitamin A can occur.

What to Do: This is unlikely to be a problem unless excessive amounts of vitamin A are being taken daily. Report any unusual symptoms (see Appendix 18) to your doctor, nurse or pharmacist.

E-1

Drug: **Edetate Disodium (EDTA)**

Food: Copper, iron, magnesium, zinc

Outcome: EDTA and these nutrients form a complex which results in nutrient loss and decreased drug action.

What to Do: Eat a balanced diet. Your doctor will recommend dietary changes if they are indicated. Notify your doctor, nurse or pharmacist if unusual symptoms appear or if your therapy does not seem to be effective.

E-2

Drug: **Enoxacin**

Food: Caffeine, coffee, tea, cola beverages

Outcome: Enoxacin interferes with the normal metabolism of caffeine. Increased caffeine levels and activity (including adverse effects) can occur.

What to Do: It is best to limit caffeine intake while on therapy.

E-3

Drug: **Enoxacin**

Food: Food in general

Outcome: Decreased drug absorption can occur.

What to Do: It is best to take this drug on an empty stomach (1 hour before or 2 hours after meals).

E-4

Drug: **Enteric-coated Medications**

Food: Food in general

Outcome: Enteric-coated drugs are designed to dissolve in the intestines rather than the stomach in order to avoid stomach distress. Food can cause these medications to remain in the stomach longer.

What to Do: It is best to take these medications on an empty stomach (i.e., 1 hour before or 2 hours after food). It is important to avoid alkaline foods (e.g., dairy products, milk) or antacids, since alkaline products can cause enteric-coated products to dissolve in the stomach, rather than the intestines.

E-5

Drug: **Ephedrine**

Food: Foods that acidify the urine (Appendix 4)

Outcome: Ephedrine is eliminated more quickly than normal in acidic urine; decreased drug effects are possible.

What to Do: Eat a balanced diet. Avoid excessive intake of these foods while on therapy. Notify your doctor, nurse or pharmacist if your therapy does not seem to be working effectively.

E-6

Drug: **Ephedrine**

Food: Foods that cause alkaline urine (Appendix 5)

Outcome: The drug is eliminated less quickly than normal in alkaline urine. Increased drug effects (including adverse drug effects) are possible.

What to Do: Eat a balanced diet. Avoid excessive intake of these foods while on therapy. Report any unusual symptoms (e.g., nervousness, restlessness, insomnia, irregular pulse, increased blood pressure) to your doctor, nurse or pharmacist.

E-7

Drug: **Ergotamine**

Food: Caffeine

Outcome: Caffeine can increased absorption of ergotamine.

What to Do: Report any unusual symptoms or side effects to your doctor, nurse or pharmacist. Consider reducing your daily caffeine intake for general health reasons.

E-8

Drug: **Erythromycin**

Food: Acidic fruits or juices, carbonated beverages, wines, syrups, tomatoes, vegetables

Outcome: Acidic foods promote premature decomposition of erythromycin, which can interfere with antibiotic effectiveness.

What to Do: It is usually best to take antibiotics with water, rather than other beverages.

E-9

Drug: **Erythromycin (enteric-coated)**

Food: Alkaline foods (e.g., milk, dairy products, vegetables)

Outcome: Alkaline foods and beverages can cause the enteric coating to dissolve in the stomach, rather than the intestines. If this happens, stomach acids can cause the drug to decompose prematurely and antibiotic effectiveness may be reduced. Also, erythromycin can be irritating to the stomach.

What to Do: It is usually best to take antibiotics with water, rather than other beverages.

E-10

Drug: **Erythromycin**

Food: Amino acids

Outcome: Erythromycin can interfere with protein synthesis.

What to Do: Antibiotic therapy is normally prescribed for less than 2 weeks, so it is unlikely that problems will develop. Your doctor will recommend dietary changes if they are indicated.

E-11

Drug: **Erythromycin**

Food: Calcium, folic acid, magnesium, vitamin B_6 (pyridoxine), vitamin B_{12}

Outcome: Erythromycin can interfere with the normal absorption, metabolism or activity of these nutrients.

What to Do: Eat a balanced diet. Antibiotic therapy is normally prescribed for less than 2 weeks, so problems are unlikely. Your doctor will recommend dietary changes if they are indicated. Report any unusual symptoms (see Appendices 12, 13, 15, 22, 23) to your doctor, nurse or pharmacist.

E-12

Drug: **Erythromycin**

Food: Food in general

Outcome: Both decreased (or delayed) and increased drug absorption have been reported. Food can reduce or delay absorption by physically interfering with absorption. It can increase absorption by causing drugs to stay in the stomach longer than normal (the stomach is the primary site of absorption for most drugs).

What to Do: It is best to take antibiotics on an empty stomach (1 hour before or 2 hours after eating). However, erythromycin antibiotics can be irritating to the stomach. Food can help to reduce this irritation. Even though food can reduce drug absorption, it probably poses little risk to therapeutic effectiveness. So, health professionals often recommend that you take these antibiotics with food. If you have questions, talk with your doctor, nurse or pharmacist.

E-13

Drug: **Estrogens**

Food: Folic acid

Outcome: Estrogens can interfere with the absorption of folic acid.

What to Do: Eat a balanced diet. Your doctor will recommend dietary changes or supplements if they are indicated. Report any unusual symptoms (see Appendix 13) to your doctor, nurse or pharmacist.

E-14

Drug: **Estrogens**

Food: Grapefruit juice

Outcome: Increased levels of some estrogen components have been reported. However, the actual effects of this observation are unknown at this time.

What to Do: Eat a balanced diet. Your doctor will recommend dietary changes or supplements if they are indicated. Report any unusual symptoms to your doctor, nurse or pharmacist.

E-15

Drug: **Estrogens**

Food: Sodium, sodium chloride (salt)

Outcome: Sodium and fluid retention can occur.

What to Do: The average American consumes 10 times the amount of sodium (i.e., salt) actually required by the body for normal functioning. So, most people are well-advised to reduce their salt intake. To help reduce your intake, eliminate salt in cooking and use it sparingly at the table (It is easier to taste salt applied directly to food at the table; cooking tends to dilute the taste of salt, so we tend to add more at the table). Also, lemon can be used as a salt substitute on appropriate foods, since it appears to be able to "fool" the taste buds.

E-16

Drug: **Estrogens**

Food: Vitamin B_6 (pyridoxine), vitamin C

Outcome: Estrogens can interfere with vitamin metabolism; vitamin deficiency is possible. Increased estrogen levels and activity (including adverse effects) have been reported with vitamin C use.

What to Do: Eat a balanced diet. Your doctor will recommend dietary changes or supplements if they are indicated. Notify your doctor, nurse or pharmacist if unusual symptoms (see Appendices 22, 24) occur or if your therapy does not seem to be working effectively.

E-17

Drug: **Ethacrynic Acid**

Food: Magnesium, potassium, zinc

Outcome: Ethacrynic acid can cause these nutrients to be eliminated from the body more quickly than normal.

What to Do: Eat a balanced diet. Your doctor will recommend dietary changes or supplements if they are indicated. Report any unusual symptoms (see Appendices 15, 16, 28) to your doctor, nurse or pharmacist.

E-18

Drug: **Ethchlorvynol**

Food: Alcohol

Outcome: This can be a dangerous mix. It can result in excessive (and possibly dangerous) sedation and depression of the central nervous system (e.g., loss of coordination, impaired judgment, decreased performance skills and alertness, slowed reaction time, increased risk of falls).

What to Do: Avoid this mix.

E-19

Drug: **Etodolac**

Food: Food in general

Outcome: Food can interfere with the absorption of etodolac. Even so, this may not be clinically significant.

What to Do: The drug is usually taken with food to reduce stomach distress. Take at the same time each day to minimize the effects of food on therapy. Notify your doctor, nurse or pharmacist if your therapy does not seem to be working effectively.

F-1

Drug: **Famotidine**

Food: Food in general

Outcome: Higher drug levels may be achieved more rapidly when famotidine is taken with food.

What to Do: No interventions are required. The drug can be taken without regard to food.

F-2

Drug: **Felodipine**

Food: Grapefruit juice

Outcome: It is thought that grapefruit juice can interfere with normal elimination of felodipine. This could result in increased drug levels and activity. The effect is less pronounced with extended release products.

What to Do: It is best to take this drug with water, rather than grapefruit juice.

F-3

Drug: **Ferrous (Iron) Sulfate**

Food: Milk

Outcome: Milk can interfere with normal iron absorption.

What to Do: It is usually best to take medications with water. Report any unusual symptoms (see Appendix 14) to your doctor, nurse or pharmacist.

F-4

Drug: **Flecanide**

Food: Smoking

Outcome: Smoking can cause flecanide to be eliminated from the body more quickly than normal; higher doses may be required for effective therapy.

What to Do: It is best not to smoke. Notify your doctor, nurse or pharmacist if your therapy does not seem to be working effectively.

F-5

Drug: **Fluoride**

Food: Milk, dairy products, calcium

Outcome: Calcium binds with fluoride and interferes with absorption.

What to Do: Avoid taking fluoride within 2 hours of these foods.

F-6

Drug: **Fluoroquinolones**

Food: Iron, zinc

Outcome: These nutrients may interfere with the absorption, drug levels and activity of some of the drugs in this category.

What to Do: Eat a balanced diet. Your doctor will recommend dietary changes if they are indicated. It is best to avoid taking the drug within 2 hours of taking supplements containing zinc. Notify your doctor, nurse or pharmacist if your therapy does not seem to be working.

F-7

Drug: **5-Fluorouracil**

Food: Vitamin B_1 (thiamine)

Outcome: The drug can interfere with the normal metabolism of thiamine to its active form; vitamin deficiency is possible.

What to Do: Eat a balanced diet. Your doctor will recommend dietary changes or supplements if they are indicated. Report any unusual symptoms (see Appendix 19) to your doctor, nurse or pharmacist.

F-8

Drug: **Fluoxetine**

Food: Alcohol

Outcome: Fluoxetine may be able to decrease alcohol consumption by problem drinkers.

What to Do: No interventions are indicated.

F-9

Drug: **Fluoxetine**

Food: L-tryptophan

Outcome: Toxicity has been reported with large doses (e.g., agitation, insomnia, aggressive behavior, headache, sweating, dizziness, agitation, aggressiveness, worsening of obsessive-compulsive disorders, nausea, vomiting). Animal studies indicate that both fluoxetine and l-tryptophan can lower blood pressure, and that the combination has an additive effect. The clinical significance of this interaction is not known.

What to Do: Eat a balanced diet. Tryptophan occurs naturally in some foods (e.g., milk), but dietary consumption should pose no problems. Avoid tryptophan supplements. Your doctor will recommend dietary changes if they are indicated. Report any unusual symptoms to your doctor, nurse or pharmacist.

F-10

Drug: **Flurazepam**

Food: Alcohol

Outcome: This can be a dangerous mix. It can result in excessive (and possibly dangerous) sedation and depression of the central nervous system (e.g., loss of coordination, impaired judgment, decreased performance skills and alertness, slowed reaction time, increased risk of falls).

What to Do: Avoid this mix.

F-11

Drug: **Fluphenazine**

Food: Coffee, tea, vitamin C (large doses)

Outcome: These beverages can decrease absorption and therapeutic effects of fluphenazine.

What to Do: Take this drug 1 hour before or 2 hours after consuming these beverages. Contact your doctor if your therapy seems ineffective.

F-12

Drug: **Fluvastatin**

Food: Carbonated beverages

Outcome: These nutrients can interfere with normal absorption and metabolism of fluvastatin.

What to Do: No interventions are indicated. The drug can be taken without regard to meals. Notify your doctor, nurse or pharmacist if your therapy does not seem to be working effectively.

F-13

Drug: **Fluvastatin**

Food: Food in general

Outcome: Food can slow the rate of absorption of the drug, but this does not appear to be clinically significant.

What to Do: No interventions are indicated. The drug can be taken without regard to meals. Notify your doctor, nurse or pharmacist if your therapy does not seem to be working effectively.

F-14

Drug: **Fluvoxamine**

Food: Smoking

Outcome: Smoking causes fluvoxamine to be metabolized more quickly than normal. This can interfere with the effectiveness of your therapy.

What to Do: Smoking is dangerous to your health. If you smoke, notify your doctor, nurse or pharmacist if your therapy does not seem to be working effectively.

F-15

Drug: **Folic Acid**

Food: Alcohol

Outcome: Alcohol can interfere with the normal absorption and activity of folic acid; vitamin depletion and deficiency are possible.

What to Do: Excessive consumption of alcohol is associated with many health problems, including nutritional deficiencies. Report any unusual symptoms (see Appendix 13) to your doctor, nurse or pharmacist.

F-16

Drug: **Fosinopril**

Food: Food in general

Outcome: Food can decrease the rate of fosinopril absorption. However, this may not be clinically significant.

What to Do: No interventions are indicated. The drug can be taken without regard to meals. Notify your doctor, nurse or pharmacist if your therapy does not seem to be working effectively.

F-17

Drug: **Furazolidone**

Food: Alcohol

Outcome: Furazolidone can interfere with the normal metabolism of alcohol. A disulfiram-type reaction (see Appendix 11) has been reported.

What to Do: Avoid alcohol while taking this drug.

F-18

Drug: **Furazolidone**

Food: Tyramine-containing foods; Pressor amines (see Appendix 7)

Outcome: Furazolidone can interfere with the normal metabolism of tyramine and related substances. This can result in a MAOI-type reaction (see Appendix 10).

What to Do: Avoid alcoholic beverages or excessive intake of these foods while on therapy. Discuss dietary precautions with your doctor, nurse or pharmacist.

F-19

Drug: **Furosemide (and other potassium-depleting diuretics)**

Food: Calcium, chlorine, magnesium, potassium, sodium, thiamine (vitamin B_1), zinc

Outcome: Diuretics increase the excretion of these nutrients; fluid and electrolyte disturbances are possible.

What to Do: Eat a balanced diet. Your doctor will recommend dietary changes or supplements if they are indicated. Report any unusual symptoms (see Appendices 12, 15, 16, 17, 19, 28,) to your doctor, nurse or pharmacist.

F-20

Drug: **Furosemide**

Food: Food in general

Outcome: Food can interfere with furosemide absorption.

What to Do: This interaction is unlikely to be a significant problem. The drug is usually taken with food to avoid stomach irritation. Notify your doctor, nurse or pharmacist if your therapy does not seem to be working effectively.

F-21

Drug: **Furoxone**

Food: Alcohol

Outcome: Furoxone can interfere with normal alcohol metabolism; a disulfiram-like reaction can occur (see Appendix 11).

What to Do: Avoid this mix.

G-1

Drug: **Ganciclovir**

Food: High-fat meals

Outcome: Fats can interfere with normal ganciclovir absorption.

What to Do: Take as directed at the same time each day in order to avoid the impact that food might have on therapy.

G-2

Drug: **Gemfibrozil**

Food: Cholesterol, fat, iron, vitamins (e.g., A, B_{12}, D, E, K)

Outcome: Gemfibrozil can interfere with the normal absorption and activity of these nutrients.

What to Do: Eat a balanced diet. Your doctor will recommend dietary changes and supplements if they are indicated. Report any unusual symptoms (see Appendices 18, 23, 25, 26, 27) to your doctor, nurse or pharmacist.

G-3

Drug: **Gentamicin**

Food: Calcium, magnesium, potassium

Outcome: Gentamicin can result in depletion of these nutrients.

What to Do: Antibiotic therapy usually lasts for relatively short time periods, so this interaction is not usually a problem. Your doctor will recommend dietary changes or supplements if they are indicated. Report any unusual symptoms (see Appendices 12, 15, 16) to your doctor, nurse or pharmacist.

G-4

Drug: **Glibenclamide**

Food: Alcohol

Outcome: Glibenclamide can interfere with normal alcohol metabolism; a disulfiram-type reaction is possible (see Appendix 11).

What to Do: Avoid this mix.

G-5

Drug: **Glipizide**

Food: Alcohol

Outcome: Alcohol can prolong the activity of the glipizide. A disulfiram-type reaction has been reported with some drugs of this type (see Appendix 11).

What to Do: It is best to avoid alcohol while on therapy without first consulting a health professional.

G-6

Drug: **Glipizide**

Food: Food in general

Outcome: Food can interfere with normal absorption of glipizide.

What to Do: This drug is most effective when taken on an empty stomach. However, it can be taken with food if stomach distress is a problem.

G-7

Drug: **Glucocorticoids**

Food: Calcium, vitamin D

Outcome: These drugs have a negative effect on calcium and vitamin D levels and activity in the body. Long-term use can result in significant bone loss (osteoporosis).

What to Do: Eat a balanced diet. Your doctor will recommend dietary changes or supplements if they are needed. Report any unusual symptoms (see Appendix 12) to your doctor, nurse or pharmacist.

G-8

Drug: **Glucocorticoids**

Food: Potassium

Outcome: Decreased potassium levels can occur.

What to Do: Eat a balanced diet. Your doctor will recommend dietary changes or supplements if they are indicated. Report any unusual symptoms (see Appendix 16) to your doctor, nurse or pharmacist.

G-9

Drug: **Glutethimide**

Food: Alcohol

Outcome: This can be a dangerous mix. It can result in excessive (and possibly dangerous) sedation and depression of the central nervous system (e.g., loss of coordination, impaired judgment, decreased performance skills and alertness, slowed reaction time, increased risk of falls).

What to Do: Avoid this mix.

G-10

Drug: **Glutethimide**

Food: Vitamin D

Outcome: Decreased vitamin levels and activity have been reported.

What to Do: Eat a balanced diet. Therapy with this drug is usually short-term, so this interaction is rarely a problem. Your doctor will recommend dietary changes or supplements if they are indicated. Report any unusual symptoms (see Appendix 25) to your doctor, nurse or pharmacist.

G-11

Drug: **Griseofulvin**

Food: Alcohol

Outcome: Griseofulvin can interfere with normal alcohol metabolism; a disulfiram-type reaction (see Appendix 11) can occur.

What to Do: Avoid this mix.

G-12

Drug: **Griseofulvin**

Food: Food in general, high-fat foods (e.g., butter, margarine, bacon, pork)

Outcome: Fats increase the absorption of griseofulvin.

What to Do: Griseofulvin is usually taken with food to maximize therapy.

G-13

Drug: **Griseofulvin**

Food: Low-fat diet

Outcome: Griseofulvin absorption may be decreased.

What to Do: Eat a balanced diet. Griseofulvin is usually taken with food to maximize therapy. Notify your doctor, nurse or pharmacist if your therapy does not seem to be working.

G-14

Drug: **Guanethidine**

Food: Sodium, sodium chloride (salt)

Outcome: Sodium and fluid retention.

What to Do: The average American consumes 10 times the amount of sodium (i.e., salt) actually required by the body for normal functioning. So, most people are well-advised to reduce their salt intake. To help reduce your intake, eliminate salt in cooking and use it sparingly at the table (It is easier to taste salt applied directly to food at the table; cooking tends to dilute the taste of salt, so we tend to add more at the table). Also, lemon can be used as a salt substitute on appropriate foods, since it appears to be able to "fool" the taste buds.

H-1

Drug: **H2 Blockers**

Food: Alcohol

Outcome: Studies indicate that higher blood alcohol levels can occur when people drink while taking H2 blockers. The actual clinical significance of this interaction is not known.

What to Do: If you drink while taking these drugs, be aware that you may experience more sedation and loss of coordination than you would normally expect.

H-2

Drug: **Haloperidol**

Food: Coffee or tea

Outcome: These beverages can reduce absorption and therapeutic effects of haloperidol.

What to Do: Take this drug 1 hour before or 2 hours after consuming these beverages. Contact your doctor if your therapy seems ineffective.

H-3

Drug: **Heart Medications**

Food: Alcohol

Outcome: Alcohol, especially chronic use, can damage heart muscles. It may adversely affect heart efficiency in people who have heart diseases. Alcohol dilates blood vessels, which can result in drops in blood pressure, dizziness and fainting, especially when arising from a seated or lying position. Also, alcohol can mask pain that normally serves as a warning signal of problems.

What to Do: It is best to avoid alcohol use if you are being treated for heart disease without first talking with your doctor, nurse or pharmacist.

H-4

Drug: **Heart Medications**

Food: Caffeine

Outcome: Caffeine can increase heart rate and blood pressure. This could interfere with the effectiveness of heart medications.

What to Do: It is best to reduce caffeine intake while on therapy with these medications.

H-5

Drug: **Heparin**

Food: Alcohol

Outcome: An increased risk of bleeding is possible.

What to Do: It is best to avoid alcohol use while on therapy. Report any unusual symptoms to your doctor, nurse or pharmacist.

H-6

Drug: **High Blood Pressure Medications**

Food: Alcohol

Outcome: Alcohol can adversely affect heart efficiency in people who have heart diseases. Alcohol dilates blood vessels, which can result in drops in blood pressure, dizziness and fainting, especially when arising from a seated or lying position. Thus, there is an increased risk of falls. Also, alcohol can mask pain that normally serves as a warning signal of heart problems. Alcohol, especially chronic use, can damage heart muscles and can contribute to an increase in blood pressure.

What to Do: It is best to avoid alcohol use if you have high blood pressure without first consulting a health professional. Avoid getting up quickly from a seated or lying position.

H-7

Drug: **High Blood Pressure Medications**

Food: Licorice (natural), glycyrrihizic acid

Outcome: Natural licorice can cause sodium and fluid retention. This could have the effect of increasing blood pressure and interfering with the effectiveness of therapy.

What to Do: Avoid natural licorice if you are taking medications for high blood pressure. Most commercial licorice products sold in the U.S. contain artificial licorice flavoring and are not a problem for therapy.

H-8

Drug: **High Blood Pressure Medications**

Food: Salt, sodium chloride

Outcome: Fluid retention associated with salt intake can interfere with the effectiveness of therapy.

What to Do: The average American diet contains 10 times the amount of salt actually needed by the body for normal functioning. Talk with your doctor about reducing your salt intake if you have blood pressure. Using lemon on compatible foods can "fool" the taste buds so that additional salt is not missed when eating. Salting foods at the table and eliminating salt from cooking is an effective way to begin sodium reduction. Your doctor may recommend the use of salt substitutes.

H-9

Drug: **High Blood Pressure Medications**

Food: Smoking

Outcome: Smoking increases blood pressure and deprives the body of oxygen, which can contribute to heart damage.

What to Do: It is best to avoid tobacco products for general health reasons.

H-10

Drug: **High Blood Pressure Medications**

Food: Tyramine-containing foods (see Appendix 7)

Outcome: These foods can cause blood pressure to increase by causing blood vessels to constrict.

What to Do: Avoid excessive intake of these foods. Eat a balanced diet. Your doctor will recommend dietary changes if they are indicated. Notify your doctor, nurse or pharmacist regarding any unusual symptoms or if your therapy does not seem to be working effectively.

H-11

Drug: **Hydantoins**

Food: Alcohol

Outcome: Short term or periodic use of alcohol can interfere with the normal metabolism of hydantoins. This can result in increased drug activity (including adverse effects). Both alcohol and hydantoins are sedating, so that excessive sedation, loss of coordination and depression of the central nervous system can occur. Chronic alcohol use can increase metabolism of the drug, resulting in decreased drug activity and effectiveness.

What to Do: It is best to avoid alcohol use if you are being treated for seizures without first consulting with a health professional. Notify your doctor, nurse or pharmacist if unusual symptoms occur or if your therapy does not seem to be working effectively.

H-12

Drug: **Hydralazine**

Food: Food in general

Outcome: Food increases absorption of hydralazine. Higher drug levels than normal can occur.

What to Do: No interventions are indicated. This drug is normally taken with food. Report any unusual symptoms or side effects of therapy to your doctor, nurse or pharmacist.

H-13

Drug: **Hydralazine**

Food: Sodium, sodium chloride (salt)

Outcome: Sodium and fluid retention.

What to Do: The average American consumes 10 times the amount of sodium (i.e., salt) actually required by the body for normal functioning. So, most people are well-advised to reduce their salt intake. To help reduce your intake, eliminate salt in cooking and use it sparingly at the table (It is easier to taste salt applied directly to food at the table; cooking tends to dilute the taste of salt, so we tend to add more at the table). Also, lemon can be used as a salt substitute on appropriate foods, since it appears to be able to "fool" the taste buds.

H-14

Drug: **Hydralazine**

Food: Vitamin B_6 (pyridoxine)

Outcome: Hydralazine and pyridoxine can combine to form a complex which is more highly excreted in the urine; vitamin deficiency is possible.

What to Do: Eat a balanced diet. Therapy with this drug is usually short-term. Your doctor will recommend dietary changes or supplements if they are indicated. Report any unusual symptoms (see Appendix 22) to your doctor, nurse or pharmacist.

H-15

Drug: **Hydrochlorothiazide (HCTZ)**

Food: Food in general

Outcome: Both decreased and increased absorption of HCTZ have been reported.

What to Do: No interventions are indicated. This drug may be taken with food to prevent stomach distress.

H-16

Drug: **Hydrochlorothiazide (HCTZ)**

Food: Potassium

Outcome: HCTZ causes potassium to be lost in the urine.

What to Do: Patients taking these drugs are usually advised to increase their intake of foods which contain potassium (see Appendix 1). Your doctor will recommend appropriate dietary changes and supplements if they are indicated. Report any unusual symptoms (see Appendix 16) to your doctor, nurse or pharmacist.

H-17

Drug: **Hydrocortisone**

Food: Calcium, dairy products

Outcome: Decreased calcium absorption and calcium depletion are possible with high doses of hydrocortisone.

What to Do: Eat a balanced diet. Therapy with this type of drug is often short-term. Your doctor will recommend dietary changes or supplements if they are indicated. Report any unusual symptoms (see Appendix 12) to your doctor, nurse or pharmacist.

H-18

Drug: **Hypoglycemics**

Food: Alcohol

Outcome: Alcohol consumption can result in unpredictable fluctuations in blood sugar levels.

What to Do: Diabetics should avoid alcohol without first checking with a health professional.

H-19

Drug: **Hypoglycemics**

Food: Sugar, carbohydrates

Outcome: Hypoglycemics reduce levels of sugars and carbohydrates.

What to Do: These drugs are taken to decrease or control the levels of blood sugar. It is important for diabetics to follow dietary and medication instructions.

H-20

Drug: **Hypoglycemics**

Food: Vitamin B_{12}

Outcome: Hypoglycemics can interfere with the absorption of vitamin B_{12}.

What to Do: Eat a balanced diet. Your doctor will recommend dietary changes or supplements if they are indicated. Report any unusual symptoms (see Appendix 23) to your doctor, nurse or pharmacist.

I-1

Drug: **Ibuprofen**

Food: Alcohol

Outcome: Both alcohol and ibuprofen are irritating to the stomach. The risk for stomach irritation is greater when these are taken together.

What to Do: It is best to avoid alcohol while taking drugs of this type.

I-2

Drug: **Ibuprofen**

Food: Food in general

Outcome: Food can increase the time it takes for ibuprofen to start working. However, food also protects the stomach from irritation.

What to Do: The drug is usually taken with food to reduce the risk of stomach distress. If it is tolerated, the drug can be taken on an empty stomach for faster onset of action.

I-3

Drug: **Imipramine**

Food: Alcohol

Outcome: This can be a dangerous mix. It can result in excessive (and possibly dangerous) sedation and depression of the central nervous system (e.g., loss of coordination, impaired judgment, decreased performance skills and alertness, slowed reaction time, increased risk of falls). Long-term alcohol consumption can cause changes in the body so that the drug does not work as effectively as normal (e.g., decreased absorption of the drug from the intestinal tract, changes in normal metabolism or increased excretion).

What to Do: Avoid alcohol consumption while taking this drug. Contact your doctor if the drug does not appear to be working effectively.

I-4

Drug: **Imipramine**

Food: Foods that acidify the urine (see Appendix 4)

Outcome: Imipramine is excreted more quickly in acidic urine.

What to Do: Eat a balanced diet. This interaction is unlikely unless excessive amounts of these foods are consumed. Notify your doctor if your therapy does not seem to be effective.

I-5

Drug: **Imipramine**

Food: Foods that produce alkaline urine (see Appendix 5)

Outcome: Imipramine is excreted less quickly in alkaline urine.

What to Do: Eat a balanced diet. This interaction is unlikely unless excessive amounts of these foods are consumed. Notify your doctor, nurse or pharmacist if unusual symptoms or side effects occur.

I-6

Drug: **Imipramine**

Food: Riboflavin (vitamin B_2)

Outcome: Imipramine interferes with the normal metabolism of riboflavin and increases its excretion in the urine. This creates the possibility for a vitamin deficiency despite an adequate diet.

What to Do: Eat a balanced diet. Your doctor will recommend dietary changes or supplements if they are indicated. If unusual symptoms occur (see Appendix 20), notify your doctor, nurse or pharmacist.

I-7

Drug: **Indinavir**

Food: Food in general

Outcome: Food can decrease drug levels and activity.

What to Do: Indinavir should be taken on an empty stomach (1 hour before or 2 hours after meals). Drink at least 48 ounces of water daily to decrease the risk of kidney stones.

I-8

Drug: **Indomethacin**

Food: Alcohol

Outcome: Both alcohol and indomethacin are irritating to the stomach. The risk of irritation and stomach bleeding is greater when these are taken together.

What to Do: Avoid alcohol while taking this medication. Report symptoms of stomach or intestinal bleeding (i.e., blood in the stool or vomit; black, tar-like stools, "coffee grounds" vomit) or irritation (e.g., abdominal pain) to your doctor.

I-9

Drug: **Indomethacin**

Food: Applesauce

Outcome: Poor absorption of indomethacin has been reported. The actual significance is controversial and may depend upon the amount of applesauce consumed.

What to Do: It is best to take indomethacin with water.

I-10

Drug: **Indomethacin**

Food: Calcium

Outcome: Lowered calcium levels can occur.

What to Do: Eat a balanced diet. Your doctor will recommend dietary changes or supplements if they are indicated. If unusual symptoms occur (see Appendix 12), notify your doctor, nurse or pharmacist.

I-11

Drug: **Indomethacin**

Food: Food in general

Outcome: Food can delay absorption of indomethacin. However, the drug should be taken with food to avoid stomach irritation.

What to Do: It is best to take indomethacin with food to reduce the risk of stomach irritation. Report symptoms of stomach or intestinal bleeding (i.e., blood in the stool or vomit; black, tar-like stools, "coffee grounds" vomit) or irritation (e.g., abdominal pain) to your doctor.

I-12

Drug: **Indomethacin**

Food: High-protein or high-fat diets

Outcome: These foods can alter the normal absorption, distribution and excretion of indomethacin.

What to Do: It is best to take indomethacin with food to reduce the risk of stomach irritation. Notify your doctor, nurse or pharmacist if your therapy does not seem to be working effectively.

I-13

Drug: **Indomethacin**

Food: Iron

Outcome: Both indomethacin and iron are irritating to the stomach. The risk for stomach irritaiton and bleeding is greater when these are taken together. Iron losses can occur with stomach bleeding.

What to Do: Take with food to reduce the risk of stomach irritation and bleeding. Report symptoms of stomach or intestinal bleeding (i.e., blood in the stool or vomit; black, tar-like stools, "coffee grounds" vomit) or irritation (e.g., abdominal pain) to your doctor. Your doctor will recommend dietary changes or supplementation if they are indicated. Report any unusual symptoms (see Appendix 14) to your doctor, nurse or pharmacist.

I-14

Drug: **Indomethacin**

Food: Phosphate

Outcome: Decreased phosphate levels can occur.

What to Do: Eat a balanced diet. Your doctor will recommend dietary changes or supplementation if they are indicated. Report any unusual symptoms to your doctor, nurse or pharmacist.

I-15

Drug: **Indomethacin**

Food: Sodium, sodium chloride (salt)

Outcome: Sodium and fluid retention can occur.

What to Do: The average American consumes 10 times the amount of sodium (i.e., salt) actually required by the body for normal functioning. So, most people are well-advised to reduce their salt intake. To help reduce your intake, eliminate salt in cooking and use it sparingly at the table (It is easier to taste salt applied directly to food at the table; cooking tends to dilute the taste of salt, so we tend to add more at the table). Also, lemon can be used as a salt substitute on appropriate foods, since it appears to be able to "fool" the taste buds.

I-16

Drug: **Insulin**

Food: Alcohol

Outcome: Insulin activity may be increased.

What to Do: It is best to avoid alcohol use during therapy without first consulting with a health professional. Monitor blood sugar levels carefully following consumption of alcoholic beverages.

I-17

Drug: **Insulin**

Food: Smoking

Outcome: Smoking can interfere with the effectiveness of insulin.

What to Do: It is best to avoid smoking for general health reasons. If you smoke while on therapy, monitor your blood sugar levels carefully.

I-18

Drug: **Insulin**

Food: Coffee

Outcome: Increased insulin excretion has been reported.

What to Do: Diabetics should carefully monitor diet and blood sugar levels as directed by their physicians. Report any unusual symptoms that may indicate abnormal blood sugar levels.

I-19

Drug: **Iron**

Food: Caffeine, coffee, tea, cola beverages

Outcome: Iron binds with caffeine, which can result in reduced iron absorption. However, the actual clinical significance of this interaction is not known.

What to Do: Take iron supplements 1to 2 hours before or after consuming these beverages.

I-20

Drug: **Iron**

Food: Calcium, cereal, clays, dairy products, eggs, manganese, milk, starches

Outcome: These foods can interfere with normal iron absorption.

What to Do: Absorption problems can usually be avoided by taking the drug 1 hour before or 2 hours after these foods. No other interventions are usually recommended. Your doctor will recommend dietary changes or supplements if they are indicated. Report any unusual symptoms (see Appendix 14) to your doctor, nurse or pharmacist.

I-21

Drug: **Iron**

Food: Citrus fruit juices, vitamin C (ascorbic acid)

Outcome: Increased iron absorption can occur; iron toxicity is possible.

What to Do: Problems are unlikely unless the drug is consistently taken with these foods. To avoid this interaction, take the drug 1 hour before or 2 hours after consuming these foods. Report unusual symptoms (see Appendix 14) to your doctor, nurse or pharmacist.

I-22

Drug: **Iron**

Food: Vitamin E

Outcome: Decreased vitamin E absorption can occur when these two are taken together.

What to Do: No interventions are required, since vitamin E is not associated with a deficiency state. Even so, this interaction can be avoided by not taking them together (avoid taking these within 1 hour of each other).

I-23

Drug: **Iron**

Food: Zinc

Outcome: Iron supplements can interfere with normal zinc absorption.

What to Do: Avoid excessive intake of iron unless it is prescribed by a doctor. If higher doses of iron are being taken, separate zinc and iron doses by at least 1 hour. Report any unusual symptoms (see Appendices 14, 28) to your doctor, nurse or pharmacist.

I-24

Drug: **Isocarboxazid**

Food: Tyramine; foods high in pressor amines (see Appendix 7)

Outcome: A MAOI-type reaction (see Appendix 10) can occur.

What to Do: Avoid this mix. Talk to your doctor, nurse or pharmacist about dietary changes and foods to avoid while on therapy.

I-25

Drug: **Isoniazid**

Food: Alcohol

Outcome: A disulfiram-type reaction (see Appendix 11) can occur due to an interference with the normal metabolism of alcohol. This interaction may also result in drug-induced hepatitis. Finally, long-term use of alcohol can cause isoniazid to be metabolized more quickly than normal, so that it is less effective.

What to Do: Avoid this mix. Report yellowing of the skin or eyes or any other unusual symptoms (see Appendix 11) to your doctor, nurse or pharmacist immediately.

I-26

Drug: **Isoniazid**

Food: Amino acids

Outcome: Impaired protein synthesis has been reported.

What to Do: Eat a balanced diet. Your doctor will recommend dietary changes or supplements if they are indicated.

I-27

Drug: **Isoniazid**

Food: Calcium, magnesium, vitamin B_{12}

Outcome: Decreased absorption of these nutrients can occur.

What to Do: Eat a balanced diet. Your doctor will recommend dietary changes or supplements if they are indicated. Report any unusual symptoms (see Appendices 12, 15, 23) to your doctor, nurse or pharmacist.

I-28

Drug: **Isoniazid**

Food: Folic acid

Outcome: Isoniazid can interfere with normal folic acid acitivity.

What to Do: Eat a balanced diet. Your doctor will recommend dietary changes or supplements if they are indicated.

I-29

Drug: **Isoniazid**

Food: Food in general

Outcome: Food can interfere with the normal absorption of isoniazid.

What to Do: It is usually best to take isoniazid on an empty stomach (e.g., 1 hour before or 2 hours after eating). Talk with your doctor, nurse or pharmacist if the drug is irritating to your stomach.

I-30

Drug: **Isoniazid**

Food: Tyramine foods (see Appendix 7).

Outcome: A MAOI-type reaction (see Appendix 10) can occur.

What to Do: Avoid this mix. Report any unusual symptoms to your doctor, nurse or pharmacist.

I-31

Drug: **Isoniazid**

Food: Foods that contain histamines (see Appendix 1)

Outcome: Isoniazid can interfere with normal metabolism of the histamine component of these foods. This can result in severe headaches, redness and itching of eyes and face, chills, palpitations, changes in pulse rate and loose stools.

What to Do: Avoid this mix. Report these or any other unusual symptoms to your doctor, nurse or pharmacist.

I-32

Drug: **Isoniazid**

Food: Vitamin B_3 (niacin), vitamin B_6 (pyrodoxine)

Outcome: Isoniazid can interfere with the normal absorption, metabolism or activity of these nutrients. The nutrients may interfere with the therapeutic effectiveness of isoniazid.

What to Do: Eat a balanced diet. Your doctor will recommend dietary changes or supplements if they are indicated. Notify your doctor, nurse or pharmacist if your therapy does not seem to be working or if any unusual symptoms occur (see Appendices 21, 22).

I-33

Drug: **Isoniazid**

Food: Vitamin K

Outcome: Isoniazid can result in decreased bacterial synthesis of vitamin K.

What to Do: Eat a balanced diet. Your doctor will recommend dietary supplements or changes if they are indicated. Report any unusual symptoms (see Appendix 27) to your doctor, nurse or pharmacist.

I-34

Drug: **Isotretinoin (Retinoic Acid)**

Food: Vitamin A

Outcome: Increased vitamin A levels and toxicity can occur.

What to Do: Eat a balanced diet. Avoid vitamin A supplements (expecially high doses). Your doctor will recommend dietary changes or supplements if they are indicated. Report any unusual symptoms (see Appendix 18) to your doctor, nurse or pharmacist.

I-35

Drug: **Isotretinoin (Retinoic Acid)**

Food: Vitamin D

Outcome: Increased calcium levels have been reported in some patients who have been treated with this drug.

What to Do: Eat a balanced diet. Your doctor will recommend dietary changes if they are indicated. Report any unusual symptoms (see Appendix 25) to your doctor, nurse or pharmacist.

I-36

Drug: **Isradipine**

Food: Food in general

Outcome: Food may delay isradipine absorption, but this may not be clinically significant.

What to Do: Take as directed. Notify your doctor, nurse or pharmacist if your therapy does not seem to be working effectively.

I-37

Drug: **Itraconazole**

Food: Food in general

Outcome: Food increases the absorption of itraconazole.

What to Do: Itraconazole is usually taken with food to maximize therapeutic response.

K-1

Drug: **Kanamycin**

Food: Amino acids, folic acid

Outcome: Kanamycin can interfere with the normal activity of these nutrients.

What to Do: Eat a balanced diet. Your doctor will recommend dietary changes or supplements if they are indicated. Report any unusual symptoms (see Appendix 13) to your doctor, nurse or pharmacist.

K-2

Drug: **Kanamycin**

Food: Calcium, magnesium, vitamin B_{12}

Outcome: Kanamycin can interfere with absorption of these nutrients.

What to Do: Eat a balanced diet. Antibiotic therapy often lasts for 2 weeks or less. Your doctor will recommend dietary supplements or changes if they are indicated. Report any unusual symptoms (see Appendices 12, 15, 23) to your doctor, nurse or pharmacist.

K-3

Drug: **Kanamycin**

Food: Foods that alkalinize urine (see Appendix 5)

Outcome: These foods can cause kanamycin to be eliminated in the urine more quickly than normal. This could reduce the antimicrobial activity of the drug.

What to Do: Eat a balanced diet. This interaction is unlikely unless large amounts of these foods are being consumed. Notify your doctor, nurse or pharmacist if your therapy does not seem to be working effectively.

K-4

Drug: **Kanamycin**

Food: Vitamin B_6 (pyridoxine)

Outcome: Inactivation of the vitamin can occur.

What to Do: Eat a balanced diet. Antibiotic therapy usually lasts for less than 2 weeks. Your doctor will recommend dietary supplements or changes if they are indicated. Report any unusual symptoms (see Appendix 22) to your doctor, nurse or pharmacist.

L-1

Drug: **Labetalol**

Food: Food in general

Outcome: Food can increase labetalol absorption and interfere with its normal metabolism.

What to Do: No particular interventions are indicated. Notify your doctor, nurse or pharmacist if you experience any unusual symptoms or if your therapy does not seem to be working.

L-2

Drug: **Lansoprazole**

Food: Food in general

Outcome: Reduced drug levels occur when lansoprazole is taken 30 minutes after eating.

What to Do: Take as directed before eating at the same time each day in order to avoid the impact of food on therapy.

L-3

Drug: **Laxatives**

Food: Calcium, electrolytes, fats, glucose, lipids, potassium, vitamins

Outcome: Laxatives can interfere with the normal absorption of many nutrients, resulting in excessive losses and deficiencies.

What to Do: Problems are not likely to occur if laxatives are used only for short time periods. Talk to your doctor, nurse or pharmacist if you feel the need to use laxative products for more than a week or if any unusual symptoms appear (see Appendices 12, 13, 16, 18, 19-25, 27).

L-4

Drug: **Levodopa**

Food: Amino acids, high-protein diets, food in general

Outcome: Levodopa competes with amino acids for absorption into and transport within the brain. This can result in decreased drug effectiveness.

What to Do: Eat a balanced diet. Your doctor will recommend dietary restrictions or changes if they are indicated. The drug is normally taken with food in order to avoid stomach distress. It is best to take the drug at the same time each day in order to minimize the effects that food has on drug activity. Notify your doctor, nurse or pharmacist if your therapy does not seem to be working.

L-5

Drug: **Levodopa (sustained release)**

Food: Food in general

Outcome: Increased drug levels can occur.

What to Do: Take as directed at the same time each day to minimize the effects of food on therapy.

L-6

Drug: **Levodopa**

Food: High-protein foods (e.g., eggs, meat, protein supplements)

Outcome: Food can interfere with normal levodopa absorption from the intestines and cause fluctuations in therapeutic response (e.g., decreased effectiveness at the end of the day).

What to Do: This drug is normally taken with food to reduce the risk of stomach distress. Your doctor will recommend dietary changes if they are indicated. Fad diets (e.g., high-protein) have been associated with serious health problems. Notify your doctor, nurse or pharmacist if your therapy does not seem to be working effectively.

L-7

Drug: **Levodopa**

Food: Vitamin B_6 (pyridoxine); foods high in vitamin B_6 (see Appendix 2)

Outcome: The therapeutic effects of levodopa may be reduced due to increased metabolism and decreased ability of the drug to reach the brain; decreased ability to control Parkinson's disease.

What to Do: Eat a balanced diet. Avoid vitamin supplements without first consulting a health professional. Your doctor will recommend dietary changes if they are needed. Notify your doctor, nurse or pharmacist if your therapy does not seem to be effective.

L-8

Drug: **Lincomycin**

Food: Food in general

Outcome: Food can interfere with the normal absorption of lincomycin; diarrhea can occur.

What to Do: It is best to take antibiotics on an empty stomach (1 hour before or 2 hours after food). Talk with your doctor, nurse or pharmacist if you do not seem to be tolerating the drug well.

L-9

Drug: **Lincomycin**

Food: Cyclamates (sodium or calcium)

Outcome: Decreased absorption of lincomycin can occur.

What to Do: It is best to take antibiotics on an empty stomach (1 hour before or 2 hours after food). Talk with your doctor, nurse or pharmacist if your therapy does not seem to be working effectively.

L-10

Drug: **Lincomycin**

Food: Pectin

Outcome: Decreased absorption of lincomycin can occur due to binding with pectin.

What to Do: It is best to take antibiotics on an empty stomach (1 hour before or 2 hours after food). Talk with your doctor, nurse or pharmacist if your therapy does not seem to be working effectively.

L-11

Drug: **Lithium**

Food: Caffeine

Outcome: Caffeine can result in an increase in lithium tremors. One case was reported in which the tremors became worse when caffeine intake was decreased. In this particular case it was thought that the decreased intake of caffeine may have reduced the elimination of lithium by the kidneys, which resulted in an increase in lithium levels.

What to Do: Avoid excessive intake of caffeine without first talking with your doctor.

L-12

Drug: **Lithium**

Food: Food in general

Outcome: Food can increase lithium absorption. Diarrhea occurs in some individuals who have fasted before taking slow-release dosage forms of the drug. Lithium has a purgative action on an empty stomach, which results in decreased absorption. Drug reabsorption from the urine appears to be greater in individuals who have not fasted.

What to Do: The drug is normally taken with food to prevent stomach distress.

L-13

Drug: **Lithium**

Food: Foods that produce alkaline urine (see Appendix 5)

Outcome: The drug is excreted more quickly than normal in alkaline urine. This could result in decreased drug effectiveness.

What to Do: Eat a balanced diet. It is best to avoid excessive intake of these foods. Your doctor will recommend dietary changes if they are needed. Notify your doctor, nurse or pharmacist if your therapy does not seem to be working effectively.

L-14

Drug: **Lithium**

Food: Electrolytes (high intake); potassium

Outcome: Lithium excretion may be increased.

What to Do: Avoid excessive intake of electrolytes (e.g., salt substitutes) without first talking with your doctor. Notify your doctor, nurse or pharmacist if your therapy does not seem to be effective.

L-15

Drug: **Lithium**

Food: Salt (sodium chloride)

Outcome: Lithium levels appear to be related to salt intake. Low sodium levels (e.g., a salt-restricted diet) can interfere with the normal excretion of lithium and result in toxic levels (nausea, diarrhea, drowsiness, muscle weakness, lack of coordination, headache). Increased or excessive intake of salt can increase the normal excretion of the drug and decrease the effectiveness of therapy.

What to Do: A balanced diet (including salt levels) is important. Avoid fad diets and excessive intake of certain foods without first talking with your doctor. Report unusual symptoms (e.g., nausea, vomiting, abdominal pain, diarrhea, sedation, mild tremor, extreme thirst, frequent urination, enlarged thyroid gland, hypotension, seizures) to your doctor, nurse or pharmacist.

L-16

Drug: **Lomefloxacin**

Food: Food in general

Outcome: Food can interfere with lomefloxacin absorption.

What to Do: It is best to take antibiotics on an empty stomach. However, it can be taken with food to reduce the risk of stomach distress.

L-17

Drug: **Loratadine**

Food: Food in general

Outcome: Food can increase absorption, levels and activity of loratadine.

What to Do: Although the impact of food is not expected to be clinically significant, it is recommended that the drug should be taken on an empty stomach (1 hour before or 2 hours after eating).

L-18

Drug: **Lorazepam**

Food: Alcohol

Outcome: This can be a dangerous mix. It can result in excessive (and possibly dangerous) sedation and depression of the central nervous system (e.g., loss of coordination, impaired judgment, decreased performance skills and alertness, slowed reaction time, increased risk of falls). Alcohol can interfere with the normal excretion of the drug, so that drug levels and activity increase.

What to Do: Avoid this mix.

L-19

Drug: **Lovastatin**

Food: Food in general

Outcome: Lower levels of lovastatin occur when it is taken during fasting conditions. This drug is normally taken with food.

M-1

Drug: **Magnesium**

Food: Alcohol

Outcome: Alcohol can increase magnesium excretion.

What to Do: Eat a balanced diet. Avoid excessive alcohol consumption. Report any unusual symptoms (see Appendix 15) to your doctor, nurse or pharmacist.

M-2

Drug: **Manganese**

Food: Copper, iron

Outcome: Each of these substances can interfere with the normal absorption of the others.

What to Do: Eat a balanced diet.

M-3

Drug: **Mannitol**

Food: Fats

Outcome: Fat binds with mannitol and can result in decreased absorption.

What to Do: No interventions are recommended. Your doctor will recommend dietary supplements or changes if they are indicated.

M-4

Drug: **Monoamine Oxidase Inhibitors (MAOIs)**

Food: Foods high in tyramine and other pressor amines (see Appendix 7).

Outcome: Normally, the body converts tyramine-like substances in food to harmless chemicals which are excreted. However, in the presence of these drugs, tyramine is not metabolized normally and causes the release of chemicals in the body (e.g., norepinephrine) that can cause blood vessels to constrict and a tyramine or "MAOI-type reaction" (see Appendix 10) occurs.

What to Do: Avoid these foods during and for 3 weeks after therapy.

M-5

Drug: **Monoamine Oxidase Inhibitors (MAOIs)**

Food: Monosodium glutamate (MSG)

Outcome: Increased MAOI effects (see Appendix 10) have been reported.

What to Do: It is best to avoid excessive intake of foods containing MSG (e.g., Chinese food) while on therapy.

M-6

Drug: **Monoamine Oxidase Inhibitors (MAOIs)**

Food: Caffeine, coffee, tea, cola beverages

Outcome: Caffeine can enhance the effects of MAOIs.

What to Do: Avoid excessive caffeine intake while on therapy. Report any unusual symptoms (see Appendix 10) to your doctor, nurse or pharmacist.

M-7

Drug: **Monoamine Oxidase Inhibitors (MAOIs)**

Food: Tryptophan

Outcome: Deterioration of mental status has been reported.

What to Do: This interaction is unlikely to be a problem unless tryptophan is being taken in large quantities (e.g., tryptophen supplements) over time. Because tryptophan has been associated with other health problems, it is best to avoid supplemental tryptophan intake until the actual consequences of its use are better understood. Discuss dietary restrictions and changes with your doctor.

M-8

Drug: **Marijuana**

Food: Alcohol

Outcome: The combined effects of marijuana and alcohol (e.g., changes in judgement, perceptions and coordination) pose a significant risk for driving or engaging in other activities which require mental alertness and coordination. This combination has been linked to an increased risk for highway fatalities in teens.

What to Do: Avoid this mix.

M-9

Drug: **Mecamylamine**

Food: Foods that acidify the urine (see Appendix 4)

Outcome: Mecamylamine is excreted more quickly than normal in acidic urine. This can result in lower drug levels and activity.

What to Do: Eat a balanced diet. This type of interaction is unlikely unless large amounts of these foods are being consumed consistently. Contact your doctor if your therapy does not seem to be working effectively.

M-10

Drug: **Mecamylamine**

Food: Foods that produce alkaline urine (see Appendix 5)

Outcome: Mecamylamine is not excreted normally in alkaline urine. This can result in higher drug levels and activity, including side effects.

What to Do: Eat a balanced diet. This interaction is unlikely unless large amounts of these foods are being consumed consistently. Report any unusual symptoms or side effects to your doctor, nurse or pharmacist.

M-11

Drug: **Mefenamic Acid**

Food: Magnesium

Outcome: Absorption of mefenamic acid from the gastrointestinal tract is accelerated.

What to Do: No interventions are indicated.

M-12

Drug: **Meperidine**

Food: Foods that acidify the urine (see Appendix 4).

Outcome: Meperidine is excreted more quickly than normal in acidic urine. This can result in lower drug levels and activity.

What to Do: Eat a balanced diet. This type of interaction is unlikely unless large amounts of these foods are being consumed consistently. Contact your doctor if your therapy does not seem to be working effectively.

M-13

Drug: **Meperidine**

Food: Foods that produce alkaline urine (see Appendix 5).

Outcome: Meperidine is not excreted normally in alkaline urine. This can result in higher drug levels and activity, including side effects.

What to Do: Eat a balanced diet. This interaction is unlikely unless large amounts of these foods are being consumed consistently. Report any unusual symptoms or side effects to your doctor, nurse or pharmacist.

M-14

Drug: **Meprobamate**

Food: Alcohol

Outcome: Both of these drugs are sedating. Taking them together can result in exaggerated and possibly hazardous sedation and depression of the central nervous system (e.g., incoordination, impaired judgment, decreased performance skills and alertness, slowed reaction time, dizziness, increased risk of falls). In addition, alcohol can interfere with the normal metabolism and elimination of meprobamate, which can result in increased drug levels and activity (including adverse effects). Long-term alcohol consumption can increase the ability of the body to metabolize and eliminate the drug before it has a chance to work effectively.

What to Do: Avoid alcohol while taking this drug.

M-15

Drug: **Metamucil**

Food: Fats, vitamin A, vitamin D, vitamin E, vitamin K

Outcome: Fiber laxatives interfere with the absorption of these nutrients. This could result in nutrient deficiencies.

What to Do: Avoid taking fiber laxatives and nutrients at the same time (space them apart by at least an hour).

M-16

Drug: **Metformin**

Food: Alcohol

Outcome: Alcohol potentiates the effects of the drug. This could result in unpredictable effects on blood sugar.

What to Do: It is best to avoid alcohol intake while on therapy without first consulting a health professional.

M-17

Drug: **Metformin**

Food: Food in general

Outcome: Food can decrease absorption and increase the time required to achieve peak blood levels. The actual clinical significance is not known.

What to Do: The drug is usually taken with food. Take at the same time each day to avoid the impact of food on therapy.

M-18

Drug: **Methadone**

Food: Alcohol

Outcome: Both of these drugs are sedating. Taking them together can result in exaggerated and possibly hazardous sedation and depression of the central nervous system (e.g., incoordination, impaired judgment, decreased performance skills and alertness, slowed reaction time, dizziness, increased risk of falls). In addition, alcohol can interfere with the normal metabolism and elimination of the drug. Theoretically, this can result in increased drug levels and activity (including adverse effects).

What to Do: Avoid this mix.

M-19

Drug: **Methamphetamine**

Food: Foods that acidify the urine (see Appendix 4).

Outcome: Methamphetamine is excreted more quickly than normal in acidic urine. This can result in lower drug levels and activity.

What to Do: Eat a balanced diet. This type of interaction is unlikely unless large amounts of these foods are being consumed consistently. Contact your doctor, nurse or pharmacist if your therapy does not seem to be working effectively.

M-20

Drug: **Methamphetamine**

Food: Foods that produce alkaline urine (see Appendix 5).

Outcome: Methamphetamine is excreted less quickly than normal in alkaline urine. This can result in higher drug levels and activity (including adverse effects).

What to Do: Eat a balanced diet. This type of interaction is unlikely unless large amounts of these foods are being consumed consistently. Contact your doctor, nurse or pharmacist if you experience unusual symptoms or side effects.

M-21

Drug: **Methenamine**

Food: Foods that produce alkaline urine (see Appendix 5).

Outcome: Alkaline urine interferes with the normal conversion of the drug to its active metabolite. The drug is not as effective in alkaline urine.

What to Do: Eat a balanced diet. Avoid excessive intake of these foods while on therapy. Drink ample fluids to promote adequate urine flow. Notify your doctor, nurse or pharmacist if your therapy does not seem to be working effectively.

M-22

Drug: **Methenamine**

Food: Foods that acidify the urine (see Appendix 4).

Outcome: Optimal drug activity occurs in acid urine.

What to Do: Try to avoid excessive intake of these foods. Your doctor may recommend acidic foods if they are needed to optimize therapy.

M-23

Drug: **Methotrexate**

Food: Butter, corn flakes, food in general, milk, sugar, white bread.

Outcome: These foods can interfere with the normal absorption of methotrexate.

What to Do: Eat a balanced diet. You may be instructed to take the drug with food to avoid stomach upset. Your doctor will recommend dietary changes if they are indicated. Notify your doctor, nurse or pharmacist if your therapy does not seem to be working.

M-24

Drug: **Methotrexate**

Food: Carotene, cholesterol, fats, lactose, vitamin B_{12}, d-xylose

Outcome: Methotrexate can interfere with the normal absorption of these nutrients.

What to Do: Eat a balanced diet. Your doctor will recommend dietary changes or supplements if they are indicated. Report any unusual symptoms to your doctor, nurse or pharmacist (see Appendix 23).

M-25

Drug: **Methotrexate**

Food: Folic acid

Outcome: The drug interferes with the normal absorption, metabolism and activity of folic acid; folic acid depletion and deficiency is possible. Folic acid supplements can alter the normal drug response.

What to Do: Eat a balanced diet. Your doctor will recommend dietary changes or supplements if they are indicated. Notify your doctor, nurse or pharmacist if unusual symptoms occur (see Appendix 13).

M-26

Drug: **Methotrexate**

Food: Para-aminobenzoic acid (PABA)

Outcome: PABA can displace the drug from its normal binding sites, which can result in increased drug levels and activity, including adverse effects.

What to Do: Eat a balanced diet. Your doctor will recommend dietary changes if they are indicated. Notify your doctor, nurse or pharmacist if any unusual symptoms or side effects occur.

M-27

Drug: **Methylcellulose (and other bulk fiber laxatives)**

Food: Calcium, iron, magnesium, zinc

Outcome: These laxatives can interfere with the normal absorption of these nutrients; deficiencies are possible.

What to Do: Eat a balanced diet. Take food or nutrients 2 hours before or after taking these laxatives. Report unusual symptoms (see Appendices 12, 14, 15, 28) to your doctor, nurse or pharmacist.

M-28

Drug: **Methyldopa**

Food: Food in general, high-protein diets

Outcome: Food can interfere with the normal absorption of methyldopa.

What to Do: It is usually best to take medications on an empty stomach (1 hour before or 2 hours after eating) unless they cause stomach distress.

M-29

Drug: **Methyldopa**

Food: Neutral amino acids

Outcome: The food can interfere with the normal ability of the drug to reach the brain.

What to Do: Eat a balanced diet. Your doctor will recommend dietary changes if they are indicated. Notify your doctor, nurse or pharmacist if your therapy does not seem to be effective.

M-30

Drug: **Methyldopa**

Food: Sodium (salt)

Outcome: Sodium and fluid retention can occur.

What to Do: The average American consumes 10 times the amount of sodium (i.e., salt) actually required by the body for normal functioning. So, most people are well-advised to reduce their salt intake. To help reduce your intake, eliminate salt in cooking and use it sparingly at the table. It is easier to taste salt applied directly to food at the table. Cooking tends to dilute the taste of salt, so we tend to add more at the table. Also, lemon can be used as a salt substitute on appropriate foods, since it appears to be able to "fool" the taste buds.

M-31

Drug: **Methyldopa**

Food: Vitamin B_{12}

Outcome: Decreased B_{12} levels and deficiency can occur.

What to Do: Eat a balanced diet. Your doctor will recommend dietary changes or supplements if they are indicated. Report any unusual symptoms to your doctor, nurse or pharmacist (see Appendix 23).

M-32

Drug: **Metoclopramide**

Food: Alcohol

Outcome: Increased alcohol absorption and activity can occur. Also, alcohol is irritating to the esophagus, stomach and intestines.

What to Do: It is best to avoid alcohol during therapy. If you drink, do so only in moderation and be aware that the effects of alcohol may occur with fewer drinks than you would normally anticipate.

M-33

Drug: **Metoprolol**

Food: Food in general

Outcome: Increased absorption and activity of metoprolol can occur.

What to Do: Take at the same time each day with regard to food in order to avoid the effects which food might have on drug activity. It is usually best to take this medication on an empty stomach unless stomach irritation occurs. Report unusual side effects or symptoms to your doctor, nurse or pharmacist.

M-34

Drug: **Metronidazole**

Food: Alcohol

Outcome: The drug can interfere with the normal metabolism of alcohol; a disulfiram-type reaction (see Appendix 11) can occur.

What to Do: Avoid this mix.

M-35

Drug: **Metronidazole**

Food: Food in general

Outcome: Delayed absorption of metronidazole can occur.

What to Do: It is usually best to take this drug with food to avoid stomach distress.

M-36

Drug: **Mexiletine**

Food: Foods that acidify the urine (see Appendix 4).

Outcome: Unpredictable changes can occur in acid urine. The drug may be excreted more quickly than normal, which could result in decreased drug effects.

What to Do: Eat a balanced diet. It is probably best to avoid excessive intake of these foods while on therapy. There is a lack of general agreement regarding the actual clinical significance of this interaction. Your doctor will recommend dietary changes if they are indicated. Notify your doctor if your therapy does not seem to be workingly effectively.

M-37

Drug: **Mexiletine**

Food: Foods that produce alkaline urine (see Appendix 5)

Outcome: Unpredictable changes can occur in acid urine. The drug may be excreted more slowly than normal, resulting in increased activity and effects (including adverse drug effects).

What to Do: Eat a balanced diet. It is probably best to avoid excessive intake of these foods while on therapy. There is a lack of general agreement regarding the actual clinical significance of this interaction. Your doctor will recommend dietary changes if they are indicated. Report any unusual side effects or symptoms to your doctor, nurse or pharmacist.

M-38

Drug: **Mexiletine**

Food: Caffeine

Outcome: Mexiletine reduces the elimination of caffeine and increases the risk for adverse effects.

What to Do: Reduce caffeine intake. Report any unusual symptoms or side effects to your doctor, nurse or pharmacist (e.g., inability to sleep, rapid or irregular pulse, increased blood pressure, nervousness, agitation, nausea, vomiting, diarrhea, tremors).

M-39

Drug: **Mexiletine**

Food: Food in general

Outcome: Food can interfere with the normal absorption of Mexiletine.

What to Do: The drug is usually taken with food to avoid stomach irritation. Your doctor will recommend dietary changes if they are indicated. Notify your doctor, nurse or pharmacist if your therapy does not seem to be effective.

M-40

Drug: **Midazolam**

Food: Grapefruit juice

Outcome: Increased midazolam blood levels and activity (including adverse effects) can occur.

What to Do: It is best to take medications with water, rather than other beverages. Report any unusual symptoms (e.g., sedation) to your doctor, nurse or pharmacist.

M-41

Drug: **Mineral Oil**

Food: Calcium, carotene, lipids, phosphorus, potassium, vitamin A, vitamin D, vitamin E, vitamin K

Outcome: Mineral oil interferes with the absorption of these nutrients. Nutrient deficiencies are possible with excessive or chronic use of mineral oil.

What to Do: It is best to take mineral oil on an empty stomach. Talk to a health professional before using mineral oil. Laxatives should only be used on an occasional basis and should never be used for more than a week without consulting a doctor, nurse or pharmacist. Even when a laxative is needed, mineral oil is not a good first choice for self-care practices.

M-42

Drug: **Misoprostol**

Food: Food in general

Outcome: Lower misoprostol levels occur when it is taken with food. This could result in decreased effectiveness of therapy.

What to Do: Take the drug as directed at the same time each day in order to minimize the impact of food on therapy.

M-43

Drug: **Moricizine**

Food: Food in general

Outcome: Food interferes with the rate of drug absorption, but the overall extent of absorption is not altered.

What to Do: No interventions are indicated.

M-44

Drug: **Morphine**

Food: High-protein or high-fat foods

Outcome: Increased levels and activity of morphine are possible, although the actual clinical significance is unknown.

What to Do: This interaction is unlikely to occur unless these foods are consumed in excessive or continuous amounts. Your doctor will recommend dietary changes if they are indicated. Report any unusual symptoms or side effects to your doctor, nurse or pharmacist.

M-45

Drug: **Moxalactam**

Food: Alcohol

Outcome: Acute alcohol intolerance (a disulfiram-type reaction, see Appendix 11) can occur because the drug interferes with the normal metabolism of alcohol. The reaction begins within 30 minutes after alcohol ingestion and subsides within 1 to several hours later. The reaction can occur up to 3 days after the last dose of the antibiotic is taken.

What to Do: Avoid this mix. Do not drink during therapy or for 72 hours after therapy has been completed.

M-46

Drug: **Moxalactam**

Food: Vitamin K

Outcome: Depleted vitamin levels can occur.

What to Do: Antibiotics are usually taken for less than 2 weeks, so it is unlikely that this interaction will cause problems. Your doctor will recommend dietary changes if they are necessary. Report any unusual symptoms (see Appendix 27) to your doctor, nurse or pharmacist.

N-1

Drug: **Nafcillin**

Food: Food in general

Outcome: Food can interfere with the normal absorption of nafcillin.

What to Do: It is usually best to take antibiotics on an empty stomach (1 hour before or 2 hours after eating). If the drug seems to irritate your stomach (e.g. nausea, vomiting, abdominal pain), contact your doctor, nurse or pharmacist.

N-2

Drug: **Nalidixic Acid**

Food: Foods that produce alkaline urine (see Appendix 5).

Outcome: The drug is excreted more quickly than normal in alkaline urine. This could result in decreased effectiveness of therapy.

What to Do: Eat a balanced diet. This interaction is unlikely unless excessive amounts of these foods are consumed. Your doctor will recommend dietary changes if they are indicated. Notify your doctor, nurse or pharmacist if your therapy does not seem to be working effectively.

N-3

Drug: **Nalidixic Acid**

Food: Foods that acidify the urine (see Appendix 4).

Outcome: The drug is not excreted normally in acidic urine. This can result in higher drug levels and activity (including adverse effects).

What to Do: Eat a balanced diet. This interaction is unlikely unless excessive amounts of these foods are consumed. Your doctor will recommend dietary changes if they are indicated. Notify your doctor, nurse or pharmacist if you experience unusual symptoms or side effects.

N-4

Drug: **Narcotics**

Food: Folic acid

Outcome: An increased need for folic acid can occur.

What to Do: Significant problems are unlikely, since narcotics are not usually taken continuously for long time periods. Your doctor will recommend dietary changes or supplements if they are indicated. Notify your doctor, nurse or pharmacist if you notice unusual symptoms (see Appendix 13).

N-5

Drug: **Narcotics**

Food: Foods that acidify the urine (see Appendix 4).

Outcome: Narcotics are excreted more quickly than normal in acid urine. This can result in decreased levels and activity.

What to Do: Eat a balanced diet. This interaction is unlikely unless excessive amounts of these foods are consumed. Your doctor will recommend dietary changes if they are indicated. Notify your doctor, nurse or pharmacist if your therapy seems not to be effective.

N-6

Drug: **Narcotics**

Food: Foods that produce alkaline urine (see Appendix 5).

Outcome: The drug is not excreted normally in alkaline urine. Increased drug activity (including adverse effects) can occur.

What to Do: Eat a balanced diet. This interaction is unlikely unless excessive amounts of these foods are consumed. Your doctor will recommend dietary changes if they are indicated. Report unusual symptoms or side effects to your doctor, nurse or pharmacist.

N-7

Drug: **Narcotics**

Food: Iron, vitamin C

Outcome: An increased need for these nutrients can occur.

What to Do: Significant problems are unlikely, since narcotics are not usually taken continuously for long time periods. Your doctor will recommend dietary changes or supplements if they are indicated. Notify your doctor, nurse or pharmacist if you notice unusual symptoms (see Appendices 14, 24).

N-8

Drug: **Nasal Decongestants**

Food: Foods that acidify the urine (see Appendix 4)

Outcome: These drugs are excreted more quickly than normal in acid urine. This could result in lower drug levels, drug activity and decreased effectiveness.

What to Do: Eat a balanced diet. Your doctor will recommend dietary changes if they are indicated. Notify your doctor, nurse or pharmacist if your therapy does not seem to be working effectively.

N-9

Drug: **Nasal Decongestants**

Food: Foods that alkalinize the urine (see Appendix 5)

Outcome: These drugs are excreted more slowly than normal in alkaline urine. This could result in higher drug levels and drug activity, including adverse drug effects.

What to Do: Eat a balanced diet. Your doctor will recommend dietary changes if they are indicated. Report any unusual side effects or symptoms to your doctor, nurse or pharmacist.

N-10

Drug: **Neomycin**

Food: Amino acids

Outcome: The drug can interfere with the normal role of amino acids in protein synthesis.

What to Do: Antibiotics are usually taken for short time periods, so it is unlikely that this interaction will cause problems. Your doctor will recommend dietary changes if they are necessary. Report any unusual symptoms to your doctor, nurse or pharmacist.

N-11

Drug: **Neomycin**

Food: Calcium, carbohydrates, carotene, cholesterol, electrolytes, fats, fatty acids, folic acid, iron, lactose, sucrose (sugar), magnesium, nitrogen, potassium, sodium, triglycerides, vitamins (e.g., A, B_{12}, D, K), d-xylose.

Outcome: Neomycin can increase excretion or interfere with normal absorption of these nutrients. This could result in deficiencies.

What to Do: Eat a balanced diet. Antibiotics are usually taken for short time periods, so it is unlikely that this interaction will cause problems. Your doctor will recommend dietary changes if they are necessary. Report any unusual symptoms to your doctor, nurse or pharmacist.

N-12

Drug: **Neomycin**

Food: Vitamin B_6 (pyridoxine)

Outcome: Inactivation of the vitamin can occur.

What to Do: Eat a balanced diet. Antibiotics are usually taken for short time periods, so it is unlikely that this interaction will cause problems. Your doctor will recommend dietary changes if they are necessary. Report any unusual symptoms to your doctor, nurse or pharmacist (see Appendix 22).

N-13

Drug: **Neomycin**

Food: Vitamin K

Outcome: Neomycin results in impaired absorption and destruction of the bacteria that normally synthesize vitamin K. This can result in a vitamin deficiency.

What to Do: Eat a balanced diet. Antibiotics are usually taken for short time periods, so it is unlikely that this interaction will cause problems. Your doctor will recommend dietary changes if they are necessary. Report any unusual symptoms to your doctor, nurse or pharmacist (see Appendix 27).

N-14

Drug: **Neuroleptic Agents (e.g., fluphenazine, haloperidol)**

Food: Coffee, tea

Outcome: These foods can interfere with the normal absorption of these drugs. This can result in variations in drug levels and therapeutic activity.

What to Do: It is generally best to avoid excessive caffeine intake.

N-15

Drug: **Nicardipine**

Food: Grapefruit juice

Outcome: Increase absorption and decreased elimination of nicardipine has been reported. Increased levels and activity of the drug are possible (including adverse drug effects).

What to Do: It is best to take this medication with water. Report any unusual symptoms (e.g., flushing, headache, rapid pulse, lowered blood pressure).

N-16

Drug: **Nicotine, Nicotine Gum**

Food: Acidic foods (e.g., cola beverages, coffee, fruit juices, tea)

Outcome: Oral nicotine absorption depends upon the acidity of saliva. Acidic substances consumed at the same time as nicotine can interfere with nicotine absorption. Many smokers may inadvertently interfere with their therapy, especially in the morning when the craving for cigarettes is strong and the tendency to consume these beverages is high.

What to Do: Avoid these foods within 1 to 2 hours of chewing the gum.

N-17

Drug: **Nicotine, Nicotine Gum**

Food: Foods that acidify the urine (see Appendix 4)

Outcome: Nicotine is excreted more quickly than normal in acid urine.

What to Do: Eat a balanced diet. This interaction is unlikely unless excessive quantities of these foods are consumed. Notify your doctor, nurse or pharmacist if your therapy does not seem to be effective.

N-18

Drug: **Nicotine, Nicotine Gum**

Food: Foods that produce alkaline urine (see Appendix 5)

Outcome: The drug is not excreted normally in alkaline urine. This can result in increased drug levels and activity (including adverse effects).

What to Do: Eat a balanced diet. This interaction is unlikely unless excessive quantities of these foods are consumed. Notify your doctor, nurse or pharmacist if unusual symptoms or side effects occur.

N-19

Drug: **Nifedipine**

Food: Food in general (especially low-fat meals)

Outcome: Slows the rate, but not the extent of nifedipine absorption.

What to Do: Eat a balanced diet. The drug can be taken without regard to meals.

N-20

Drug: **Nifedipine**

Food: Grapefruit juice

Outcome: Increase absorption and decreased elimination of nifedipine has been reported. Increased levels and activity of the drug are possible (including adverse drug effects).

What to Do: It is best to take this medication with water. Report any unusual symptoms (e.g., flushing, headache, rapid pulse, lowered blood pressure) to your doctor, nurse or pharmacist.

N-21

Drug: **Nifedipine**

Food: Minerals

Outcome: Minerals can bind with nifedipine and interfere with normal drug levels, activity and effectiveness.

What to Do: In general, nifedipine can be taken with food. However, it is probably best to avoid taking it with mineral supplements (i.e., take the drug 1 to 2 hours before or after taking mineral supplements).

N-22

Drug: **Nimodipine**

Food: Grapefruit juice

Outcome: Increased absorption, drug levels and activity

(including adverse drug effects) of nimodipine can occur.

What to Do: It is best to take medications with water, rather than other fluids. Report any unusual side effects (e.g., flushing, headache, rapid pulse, hypotension) to your doctor, nurse or pharmacist.

N-23

Drug: **Nitrates**

Food: Alcohol

Outcome: Low blood pressure (possibly severe) can occur. This can result in dizziness when arising quickly from a seated or lying position; cardiovascular collapse can occur in extreme cases.

What to Do: Avoid this mix.

N-24

Drug: **Nitrofurantoin**

Food: Alcohol

Outcome: Nitrofurantoin can interfere with the normal metabolism of alcohol and result in a disulfiram-type reaction (see Appendix 11).

What to Do: Avoid this mix.

N-25

Drug: **Nitrofurantoin**

Food: Food in general

Outcome: Food causes nitrofurantoin to remain in the stomach longer. This delay permits it to dissolve in the stomach before it passes into the small intestines. As a result, drug absorption, levels and activity are increased.

What to Do: Nitrofurantoin is normally taken with food to avoid stomach distress and because food enhances the absorption and effectiveness of therapy.

N-26

Drug: **Nitrofurantoin**

Food: Foods that acidify the urine (see Appendix 4).

Outcome: Nitrofurantoin has increased antimicrobial activity in acid urine.

What to Do: Eat a normal diet and avoid excessive intake of these foods. Your doctor will recommend dietary changes if they are indicated.

N-27

Drug: **Nitrofurantoin**

Food: Foods that produce alkaline urine (see Appendix 5)

Outcome: Alkaline urine interferes with therapy.

What to Do: Eat a normal diet and avoid excessive intake of these foods. Your doctor will recommend dietary changes if they are indicated.

N-28

Drug: **Nitroglycerin**

Food: Alcohol

Outcome: Low blood pressure (possibly severe) can occur. This can result in dizziness when arising quickly from a seated or lying position; cardiovascular collapse can occur in extreme cases.

What to Do: Avoid this mix.

N-29

Drug: **Nizatidine**

Food: Food in general

Outcome: Increased nizatidine levels are theoretically possible. However, it is not thought that this will have any impact on clinical activity.

What to Do: This drug can be taken without regard to food.

N-30

Drug: **NonSteroidal Anti-Inflammatory Agents (NSAIDs)**

Food: Alcohol

Outcome: These drugs and alcohol are irritating to the stomach.

Taken together, they can result in stomach bleeding and even ulcers.

What to Do: It is best to avoid alcohol while taking these drugs. It you drink, do so only in moderation. Avoid taking alcohol and these medications within 2 hours of each other. Report any unusual symptoms (e.g., abdominal pain; black, tar-like feces; black specks in vomit) to your doctor, nurse or pharmacist.

N-31

Drug: **NonSteroidal Anti-Inflammatory Drugs (NSAIDs)**

Food: Caffeine, coffee, tea, fruit juices

Outcome: These drugs and nutrients are irritating to the stomach and can result in an increased risk of stomach irritation and bleeding.

What to Do: It is best to avoid taking these drugs at the same time that these nutrients are consumed. Take these medications with a full glass of water.

N-32

Drug: **NonSteroidal Anti-Inflammatory Agents (NSAIDs)**

Food: Food in general

Outcome: Delayed absorption of the drug.

What to Do: These drugs are normally taken with food to avoid stomach distress. Delays in absorption of these drugs will not usually affect overall therapeutic effectiveness.

N-33

Drug: **Norfloxacin**

Food: Calcium, iron, magnesium

Outcome: Norfloxacin and these nutrients bind together, which can interfere with normal absorption of the drug; decreased drug levels and effectiveness are possible.

What to Do: It is best to take norfloxacin on an empty stomach (1 hour before or 2 hours after eating).

N-34

Drug: **Norfloxacin**

Food: Caffeine, coffee, tea, cola beverages

Outcome: Norfloxacin can interfere with the normal elimination of caffeine. This can result in increased caffeine activity (including adverse effects).

What to Do: Reduce your caffeine intake while on therapy.

N-35

Drug: **Norfloxacin**

Food: Food in general

Outcome: Decreased or delayed absorption of norfloxacin can occur.

What to Do: It is best to take this drug on an empty stomach (1 hour before or 2 hours after eating). Notify your doctor, nurse or pharmacist if stomach irritation or distress occurs.

N-36

Drug: **Nortriptyline**

Food: Foods that acidify the urine (see Appendix 4)

Outcome: Nortyiptyline excretion is increased in acid urine. In theory, this could result in decreased drug levels and therapeutic effects. However, the actual clinical significance of this interaction is unknown.

What to Do: It is probably best to avoid excessive intake of these foods while on this therapy. Eat a balanced diet. Your doctor will recommend dietary changes if they are indicated. Notify your doctor, nurse or pharmacist if your therapy does not seem to be effective.

N-37

Drug: **Nortriptyline**

Food: Foods that produce alkaline urine (see Appendix 5)

Outcome: Nortriptyline excretion is decreased in alkaline urine. In theory, this could result in increased drug levels and therapeutic effects (including side effects). However, the actual clinical significance of this interaction is unknown.

What to Do: It is probably best to avoid excessive intake of these foods while on this therapy. Eat a balanced diet. Your doctor will recommend dietary changes if they are indicated. Notify your doctor, nurse or pharmacist if you experience unusual symptoms or side effects.

N-38

Drug: **Novobiocin**

Food: Food in general

Outcome: Food can increase the time required to reach peak blood levels. However, this is not thought to cause a problem for therapy.

What to Do: It is usually best to take antibiotics on an empty stomach (e.g., 1 hour before or 2 hours after eating). However, antibiotics are often taken with food if they are irritating to the stomach or intestines. Talk with your doctor, nurse or pharmacist if you have questions about taking these drugs with food.

O-1

Drug: **Ofloxacin**

Food: Food in general

Outcome: Food interferes with normal absorption of ofloxacin. In theory, this could interfere with therapeutic effectiveness.

What to Do: It is best to take this drug on an empty stomach (1 hour before or 2 hours after eating).

O-2

Drug: **Ondansetron**

Food: Food in general

Outcome: Food can result in increased ondansetron absorption, but this is not thought to be clinically significant.

What to Do: Ondansetron can be taken without regard to food.

O-3

Drug: **Oral Contraceptives**

Food: Amino acids

Outcome: Decreased amino acid levels have been reported.

What to Do: Eat a balanced diet. Your doctor will recommend dietary changes if they are indicated.

O-4

Drug: **Oral Contraceptives**

Food: Cholesterol, triglycerides

Outcome: Increased cholesterol and triglyceride levels can occur.

What to Do: Eat a balanced diet. It is best to avoid excessive intake of cholesterol and triglycerides for better health. Your doctor will recommend specific dietary changes or they are indicated.

O-5

Drug: **Oral Contraceptives**

Food: Copper, iron

Outcome: Increased levels of these nutrients can occur.

What to Do: Eat a balanced diet. Your doctor will recommend dietary changes if they are indicated. It is best to avoid excessive intake of copper (i.e., more than the RDA) unless advised otherwise by a health professional.

O-6

Drug: **Oral Contraceptives**

Food: Folic acid

Outcome: Oral contraceptives can result in decreased folic acid levels.

What to Do: Eat a balanced diet. Your doctor will recommend dietary changes or supplements if they are indicated.

Report any unusual symptoms (Appendix 13) to your doctor, nurse or pharmacist.

O-7

Drug: **Oral Contraceptives**

Food: Glucose

Outcome: Impaired glucose tolerance can occur.

What to Do: Diabetics should monitor their glucose levels carefully while taking any medications.

O-8

Drug: **Oral Contraceptives**

Food: Manganese

Outcome: Oral contraceptives can interfere with normal absorption of manganese.

What to Do: Eat a balanced diet. Your doctor will recommend dietary changes or supplements if they are indicated.

O-9

Drug: **Oral Contraceptives**

Food: Nicotinamide, vitamins (e.g., B_1, B_2, B_6, B_{12}, C), zinc

Outcome: Depletion of these nutrients can occur.

What to Do: Eat a balanced diet. Your doctor will recommend

dietary changes or supplements if they are indicated. Report any unusual symptoms (see Appendices 19, 20, 22, 23, 24, 28) to your doctor, nurse or pharmacist.

O-10

Drug: **Oxacillin**

Food: Food in general

Outcome: Food can interfere with absorption of oxacillin.

What to Do: It is usually best to take antibiotics on an empty stomach (i.e., 1 hour before or 2 hours after eating). If stomach distress occurs, contact your doctor, nurse or pharmacist.

O-11

Drug: **Oxaprozin**

Food: Food in general

Outcome: Food interferes with normal rate, but not the overall extent of oxaprozin absorption.

What to Do: Oxaprozin is normally taken with food to prevent stomach distress.

O-12

Drug: **Oxyphenbutazone**

Food: Foods that acidify the urine (see Appendix 4).

Outcome: Oxyphenbutazone is not excreted normally in acid urine. This can result in increased drug levels and activity (including side effects).

What to Do: It is best to avoid excessive intake of these foods while on therapy. Eat a balanced diet. An appropriate intake of water helps to keep the urine more natural. Report unusual symptoms or side effects to your doctor, nurse or pharmacist.

O-13

Drug: **Oxyphenbutazone**

Food: Foods that produce alkaline urine (see Appendix 5)

Outcome: Oxyphenbutazone is excreted more quickly than normal in alkaline urine. This could result in decreased drug levels and activity.

What to Do: It is best to avoid excessive intake of these foods while on therapy. Eat a balanced diet. An appropriate intake of water helps to keep the urine more natural. Notify your doctor, nurse or pharmacist if your therapy seems not to be effective.

O-14

Drug: **Oxytetracycline**

Food: Food in general

Outcome: Decreased absorption of oxytetracycline can occur.

What to Do: It is usually best to take antibiotics on an empty stomach (i.e., 1 hour before or 2 hours after eating).

P-1

Drug: **Pain Medications (prescription)**

Food: Alcohol

Outcome: This can be a dangerous mix. It can result in excessive (and possibly dangerous) sedation and depression of the central nervous system (e.g., loss of coordination, impaired judgment, decreased performance skills and alertness, slowed reaction time, increased risk of falls).

What to Do: Avoid this mix.

P-2

Drug: **Para-Aminosalicylic Acid (PAS)**

Food: Amino acids

Outcome: Impaired protein synthesis can occur.

What to Do: Eat a healthy diet. Your doctor will recommend dietary changes or supplements if they are indicated. Notify your doctor, nurse or pharmacist if unusual symptoms occur.

P-3

Drug: **Para-Aminosalicylic Acid (PAS)**

Food: Calcium, fat, folic acid, magnesium, vitamins (e.g., B_{12})

Outcome: Impaired absorption, levels or activities of these nutrients can occur.

What to Do: Eat a healthy diet. Your doctor will recommend dietary changes or supplements if they are indicated. Report unusual symptoms (see Appendices 12, 13, 15, 23) to your doctor, nurse or pharmacist.

P-4

Drug: **Para-Aminosalicylic Acid (PAS)**

Food: Vitamin K

Outcome: Decreased bacterial synthesis of the vitamin can occur.

What to Do: Eat a healthy diet. Your doctor will recommend dietary changes or supplements if they are indicated. Report unusual symptoms (see Appendix 27) to your doctor, nurse or pharmacist.

P-5

Drug: **Penicillamine**

Food: Copper, zinc

Outcome: These nutrients can bind with the drug and interfere with normal absorption of both.

What to Do: Eat a healthy diet. Your doctor will recommend dietary changes or supplements if they are indicated. Report unusual symptoms (see Appendix 28) to your doctor, nurse or pharmacist.

P-6

Drug: **Penicillamine**

Food: Food in general

Outcome: Decreased drug absorption can occur.

What to Do: It is normally recommended that this drug be taken on an empty stomach (1 hour before or 2 hours after eating).

P-7

Drug: **Penicillamine**

Food: Iron

Outcome: Penicillamine and iron bind together. This can interfere with normal absorption of the drug and result in decreased drug effectiveness.

What to Do: It is normally recommended that this drug be taken on an empty stomach (1 hour before or 2 hours after eating).

P-8

Drug: **Penicillamine**

Food: Sodium

Outcome: Sodium excretion and sodium depletion has been reported in some patients (e.g., adrenally-suppressed patients).

What to Do: Eat a healthy diet. Your doctor will recommend dietary changes or supplements if they are indicated.

Report unusual symptoms (see Appendix 17) to your doctor, nurse or pharmacist.

P-9

Drug: **Penicillamine**

Food: Vitamin B_6 (pyridoxine)

Outcome: Increased urinary excretion of the vitamin and impaired vitamin metabolism can result in decreased vitamin activity and vitamin deficiency.

What to Do: Eat a healthy diet. Your doctor will recommend dietary changes or supplements if they are indicated. Report unusual symptoms (see Appendix 22) to your doctor, nurse or pharmacist.

P-10

Drug: **Penicillin**

Food: Acidic fruit juices, carbonated beverages, wines, sodas, syrups, acidic beverages, tomatoes, vegetables

Outcome: Acidic beverages can cause premature decomposition and inactivation of penicillin.

What to Do: It is best to take antibiotics on an empty stomach (1 hour before or 2 hours after eating). Take with water instead of other beverages. If stomach irritation occurs, contact your doctor, nurse or pharmacist.

P-11

Drug: **Penicillin**

Food: Amino acids, calcium, folic acid, iron, magnesium, potassium, vitamin B_6 (pyridoxine), vitamin B_{12}, vitamin K

Outcome: Inactivation, impaired absorption or decreased activity of these nutrients can occur.

What to Do: Eat a healthy diet. Your doctor will recommend dietary changes or supplements if they are indicated. Report any unusual symptoms (see Appendices 12, 13, 14, 15, 16, 22, 23, 27) to your doctor, nurse or pharmacist.

P-12

Drug: **Penicillin**

Food: Food in general

Outcome: Food decreases absorption and increases exposure to stomach acids, which can destroy some penicillins. Some foods may bind with penicillins and reduce absorption.

What to Do: It is best to take antibiotics on an empty stomach (1 hour before or 2 hours after eating). Take with water instead of other beverages. If stomach irritation occurs, contact your doctor, nurse or pharmacist.

P-13

Drug: **Pentamidine**

Food: Folic acid

Outcome: Pentamidine can result in folic acid deficiency and anemia.

What to Do: Eat a balanced diet. Folic acid supplements may be required for long-term therapy. Report any unusual symptoms (see Appendix 13) to your doctor, nurse or pharmacist.

P-14

Drug: **Pentazocine**

Food: Alcohol

Outcome: This can be a dangerous mix. It can result in excessive (and possibly dangerous) sedation and depression of the central nervous system (e.g., loss of coordination, impaired judgment, decreased performance skills and alertness, slowed reaction time, increased risk of falls).

What to Do: Avoid this mix.

P-15

Drug: **Pentobarbital**

Food: Alcohol

Outcome: Short term use of alcohol causes the drug to be metabolized less quickly than normal, so drug levels and activity (including adverse drug reactions) are increased. This means that therapeutic effects may occur with lower dosages. Also, both alcohol and barbiturates are sedating. This can be a dangerous mix. It can result in excessive (and possibly dangerous) sedation and depression of the central nervous system (e.g., loss of coordination, impaired judgment, decreased performance skills and alertness, slowed reaction time, increased risk of falls). With long-term alcohol use, the liver metabolizes the drug more quickly than normal. Blood levels and activity of the drug are decreased. This can cause people to use more and more of the drug in order to obtain therapeutic relief.

What to Do: Avoid this mix.

P-16

Drug: **Phenelzine**

Food: Ginseng

Outcome: Headache and tremors have been reported. Ginseng side effects include sleeplessness, nervousness, hypertension, and euphoria. An exact reaction mechanism between ginseng and phenelzine (as well as other MAOIs) is not well understood.

What to Do: It is probably best to avoid this mix.

P-17

Drug: **Phenelzine**

Food: Foods that contain tyramine (see Appendix 7)

Outcome: Phenelzine interferes with the normal metabolism of the tyramine in these foods; hypertensive crisis, intracranial bleeding, severe headache, chest pain, profuse sweating, palpitation, fast or slow pulse, visual disturbances, breathing difficulties, coma can occur.

What to Do: Avoid this mix.

P-18

Drug: **Phenobarbital**

Food: Calcium

Outcome: The drug can interefere with the normal intestinal absorption of calcium. Other reports indicate that the drug may result in metabolic changes and lowered vitamin D levels. These changes can cause decreased calcium levels and possible calcium deficiency.

What to Do: Eat a healthy diet. Your doctor will recommend dietary changes or supplements if they are indicated. Report any unusual symptoms (see Appendix 12) to your doctor, nurse or pharmacist.

P-19

Drug: **Phenobarbital**

Food: Folic acid

Outcome: Phenobarbital and food can interfere with each other. This can result in decreased drug effectiveness or lowered folic acid levels. Folic acid supplements may be required, although this could cause further interference with the normal activity of the drug (e.g., increased frequency and severity of seizures).

What to Do: Eat a healthy diet while on therapy. Your doctor will recommend dietary changes or supplements if they are indicated. Report any unusual symptoms (see Appendix 13) to your doctor, nurse or pharmacist.

P-20

Drug: **Phenobarbital**

Food: Food in general

Outcome: Decreased drug absorption can occur.

What to Do: Notify your doctor, nurse or pharmacist if your therapy does not seem to be effective.

P-21

Drug: **Phenobarbital**

Food: Foods that acidify the urine (see Appendix 4).

Outcome: Phenobarbital is not excreted normally in acid urine, so that higher than normal drug levels and activity (including adverse effects) can occur.

What to Do: Eat a balanced diet while on therapy. Your doctor will recommend dietary changes if they are indicated. An adequate intake of water helps to promote a more neutral urine.

P-22

Drug: **Phenobarbital**

Food: Foods that produce alkaline urine (see Appendix 5).

Outcome: Phenobarbital is excreted more quickly than normal in alkaline urine, resulting in lower drug levels and decreased effectiveness.

What to Do: Eat a balanced diet while on therapy. Your doctor will recommend dietary changes if they are indicated. An adequate intake of water helps to promote a more neutral urine.

P-23

Drug: **Phenobarbital**

Food: Magnesium, vitamin B_6 (pyridoxine), vitamin B_{12}, vitamin D, vitamin K, d-xylose

Outcome: Decreased levels and activity of these nutrients can occur.

What to Do: Eat a healthy diet while on therapy. Your doctor will recommend dietary changes or supplements if they are indicated. Report any unusual symptoms (see Appendices 15, 22, 23, 25, 27) to your doctor, nurse or pharmacist.

P-24

Drug: **Phenolphthalein**

Food: Calcium, fats, folic acid, glucose, minerals, potassium, sugars, vitamin D

Outcome: Stimulant laxatives interfere with the normal absorption of these and other nutrients; deficiencies can occur.

What to Do: Eat a healthy diet while on therapy. Your doctor will recommend dietary changes or supplements if they are indicated. Report any unusual symptoms (see Appendices 12, 13, 16, 25) to your doctor, nurse or pharmacist.

P-25

Drug: **Phenothiazines**

Food: Alcohol

Outcome: This can be a dangerous mix. It can result in excessive (and possibly dangerous) sedation and depression of the central nervous system (e.g., loss of coordination, impaired judgment, decreased performance skills and alertness, slowed reaction time, increased risk of falls).

What to Do: Avoid this mix.

P-26

Drug: **Phenothiazines**

Food: Coffee, tea

Outcome: Tannins in coffee and tea may bind together with phenothiazines and interfere with their normal absorption and activity.

What to Do: It is best to take the drug with water, rather than these beverages.

P-27

Drug: **Phenothiazines**

Food: Foods that acidify the urine (see Appendix 4)

Outcome: The drug is excreted more quickly than normal in acidic urine. This can result in lower than normal drug levels and activity.

What to Do: Eat a healthy diet while on therapy. This interaction is unlikely to occur unless large amounts of these foods are consumed. Your doctor will recommend dietary changes if they are indicated. An adequate intake of water helps to promote a more neutral urine.

P-28

Drug: **Phenylbutazone**

Food: Food in general

Outcome: Food can interfere with the normal absorption of phenylbutazone from the stomach and intestines.

What to Do: Phenylbutazone should be taken with food to prevent irritation and bleeding of the stomach and intestines.

P-29

Drug: **Phenylbutazone**

Food: Foods that acidify the urine (see Appendix 4).

Outcome: Phenylbutzone is not excreted normally in acidic urine. This can result in higher drug levels and activity, including adverse drug effects.

What to Do: Eat a balanced diet while on therapy. Your doctor will recommend dietary changes if they are indicated. An adequate intake of water helps to promote a more neutral urine.

P-30

Drug: **Phenylbutazone**

Food: Foods that produce alkaline urine (see Appendix 5)

Outcome: Phenylbutazone is excreted more quickly than normal in alkaline urine. This can result in lower than normal drug levels and activity.

What to Do: Eat a balanced diet while on therapy. This interaction is unlikely to occur unless large amounts of these foods are being eaten. Your doctor will recommend dietary changes if they are indicated. An adequate intake of water helps to promote a more neutral urine.

P-31

Drug: **Phenylbutazone**

Food: Sodium

Outcome: Sodium and water retention and swelling can occur.

What to Do: Eat a balanced diet while on therapy. Your doctor will recommend dietary changes if they are indicated. The average American consumes 10 times the amount of sodium (salt) required for the body for normal functioning. So, reducing salt intake is usually healthy. Using salt on food, but not in cooking, can help to reduce salt intake, while preserving flavor. Lemon can also be used as a salt substitute on appropriate foods (it appears to be able to fool the taste buds).

P-32

Drug: **Phenylpropanolamine**

Food: Caffeine, coffee, cola beverages, tea

Outcome: Caffeine levels may be increased, resulting in increased drug activity (including adverse effects).

What to Do: It is best to limit caffeine intake while on therapy.

P-33

Drug: **Phenytoin**

Food: Alcohol

Outcome: Both alcohol and phenytoin can cause sedation. When taken together, the sedation can be more extreme than expected. Long-term alcohol use can interfere with the normal effectiveness of the drug.

What to Do: Avoid this mix. Excessive or long-term alcohol consumption can be hazardous to health.

P-34

Drug: **Phenytoin**

Food: Calcium

Outcome: Phenytoin can interfere with normal vitamin D levels and calcium absorption from the intestines. This could result in decreased calcium levels and activity in the body; calcium deficiency is possible.

What to Do: Eat a balanced diet. Your doctor will recommend dietary changes or supplements if they are indicated.

Report any unusual symptoms (see Appendices 12, 25) to your doctor, nurse or pharmacist.

P-35

Drug: **Phenytoin**

Food: Cantaloupe, dark green leafy vegetables, folic acid, liver, navy beans, nuts, oranges, whole wheat products, yeast

Outcome: Decreased drug absorption can occur.

What to Do: Phenytoin is usually taken with food to reduce the risk of stomach upset. Notify your doctor, nurse or pharmacist if your therapy does not seem to be working.

P-36

Drug: **Phenytoin**

Food: Charcoal-broiled food

Outcome: These foods appear to be able to increase normal phenytoin metabolism. This could result in lower than normal levels of the drug in the blood and reduced effectiveness.

What to Do: Eat a balanced diet while on therapy. Your doctor will recommend dietary changes if they are indicated. Notify your doctor, nurse or pharmacist if your therapy does not appear to be effective.

P-37

Drug: **Phenytoin**

Food: Food in general

Outcome: Food causes phenytoin to remain in the stomach longer, so absorption is increased. This can result in higher levels of the drug in the blood.

What to Do: The drug is normally taken with food in order to reduce stomach upset.

P-38

Drug: **Phenytoin**

Food: Folic acid

Outcome: Both interfere with each other. Phenytoin can interfere with normal folic acid absorption. This can result in deficiency. Folic acid can reduce effectiveness of phenytoin, so that the frequency and severity of seizures are increased. To avoid deficiency folic acid supplementation is sometimes attempted. However, this can reduce effectiveness of the drug even more.

What to Do: Eat a healthy diet. Your doctor will recommend dietary changes or supplements if they are indicated. Notify your doctor, nurse or pharmacist if your therapy does not appear to be effective, or if unusual symptoms occur (see Appendix 13).

P-39

Drug: **Phenytoin**

Food: MSG (monosodium glutamate)

Outcome: Increased MSG absorption and adverse effects have been reported (e.g., weakness, numbness in the back of the neck, palpitations).

What to Do: Eat a healthy diet while on therapy. Your doctor will recommend dietary changes if they are indicated. Notify your doctor, nurse or pharmacist if unusual symptoms occur.

P-40

Drug: **Phenytoin**

Food: Nasogastric feeding products and vanilla pudding that contain caseinates, corn oil, starch, coconut oil and carrageenan.

Outcome: Lower than normal blood levels of phenytoin have been reported, despite seemingly adequate phenytoin doses. In theory, this could result in less effective drug activity.

What to Do: Eat a healthy diet while on therapy. Your doctor will recommend dietary changes if they are indicated. Notify your doctor, nurse or pharmacist if your therapy does not seem to be effective.

P-41

Drug: **Phenytoin**

Food: Vitamins (e.g., B_{12}, C, D, K), minerals, d-xylose

Outcome: Depletion, deficiency or impaired activity of these nutrients has been reported.

What to Do: Eat a healthy diet while on therapy. Your doctor will recommend dietary changes or supplements if they are indicated. Notify your doctor, nurse or pharmacist if unusual symptoms occur (see Appendices 12, 15, 23, 24, 25, 27, 28, etc.).

P-42

Drug: **Phenytoin**

Food: Vitamin B_6 (pyridoxine)

Outcome: The vitamin appears to decrease phenytoin levels and activity; decreased drug effectiveness is possible.

What to Do: Eat a healthy diet. Your doctor will recommend dietary changes if they are indicated. Notify your doctor, nurse or pharmacist if your therapy does not seem to be working effectively.

P-43

Drug: **Piroxicam**

Food: Alcohol

Outcome: Both are irritating to the stomach and intestines. When taken together, the irritation is likely to be more extreme.

What to Do: Avoid this mix.

P-44

Drug: **Piroxicam**

Food: Food in general

Outcome: Delayed piroxicam absorption can occur.

What to Do: This drug is normally taken with food to avoid stomach distress.

P-45

Drug: **Polymixin**

Food: Amino acids, calcium, folic acid, magnesium, vitamin B_6 (pyridoxine), vitamin B_{12}

Outcome: Interference with normal absorption, blood levels or activity of these nutrients can occur.

What to Do: Eat a healthy diet while on therapy. Your doctor will recommend dietary changes or supplements if they are indicated. Notify your doctor, nurse or pharmacist if unusual symptoms occur (see Appendices 12, 13, 15, 22, 23).

P-46

Drug: **Potassium**

Food: Food in general

Outcome: Delayed potassium absorption can occur.

What to Do: Potassium products are normally taken with food in order to avoid stomach distress.

P-47

Drug: **Potassium (e.g., Salt Substitutes)**

Food: Foods high in potassium (see Appendix 1).

Outcome: Increased potassium levels can occur.

What to Do: Eat a balanced diet. Follow dietary guidelines provided by your doctor. In general, never take potassium supplements unless advised to do so by a health professional. Report unusual symptoms (see Appendix 16) to your doctor, nurse or pharmacist.

P-48

Drug: **Potassium**

Food: Milk

Outcome: It has been reported that milk reacts with potassium solutions. However, a specific outcome is not proposed.

What to Do: Nothing is indicated.

P-49

Drug: **Potassium Chloride**

Food: Vitamin B_{12}

Outcome: In theory, potassium could interfere with normal absorption of the vitamin, resulting in decreased vitamin levels and deficiency.

What to Do: Eat a balanced diet. Vitamin B_{12} deficiency as a result of this interaction is rare and would take several years to develop.

P-50

Drug: **Pravastatin**

Food: Food in general

Outcome: Food can theoretically interfere with normal pravastatin levels, but its overall effectiveness does not seem to be significantly affected.

What to Do: The drug can be taken without regard to meals.

P-51

Drug: **Primidone**

Food: Folic acid, vitamin B_{12}, d-xylose

Outcome: Primidone can interfere with the normal absorption, metabolism or activity of these nutrients; deficiency is possible.

What to Do: Eat a healthy diet while on therapy. Your doctor will recommend dietary changes or supplements if they are indicated. Notify your doctor, nurse or pharmacist if unusual symptoms occur (see Appendices 13, 23).

P-52

Drug: **Probenecid**

Food: Riboflavin (vitamin B_2)

Outcome: Decreased excretion of vitamin has been reported.

What to Do: Eat a healthy diet while on therapy. Your doctor will recommend dietary changes if they are indicated.

P-53

Drug: **Probenecid**

Food: Urate-rich diets

Outcome: Decreased drug effectiveness can occur.

What to Do: Eat a healthy diet while on therapy. Your doctor will recommend dietary changes if they are indicated. Notify your doctor, nurse or pharmacist if your therapy seems not to be effective.

P-54

Drug: **Procainamide**

Food: Alcohol

Outcome: Increased procainamide excretion and reduced effectiveness has been reported. However, the actual clinical significance of this interaction is unclear.

What to Do: Avoid mixing drugs and alcohol. Discuss alcohol consumption with your doctor, nurse or pharmacist.

P-55

Drug: **Procarbazine**

Food: Alcohol

Outcome: Procarbazine can interfere with normal alcohol metabolism; a disulfiram-type reaction is possible (see Appendix 11).

What to Do: Avoid this mix.

P-56

Drug: **Procarbazine**

Food: Foods high in tyramine and other pressor amines.

Outcome: Procarbazine interferes with the normal metabolism of the chemicals in these foods. This can result in a MAOI-type of reaction (see Appendix 10).

What to Do: Avoid this mix.

P-57

Drug: **Propantheline**

Food: Food in general

Outcome: Decreased absorption of the propantheline can occur.

What to Do: The drug is usually taken with food.

P-58

Drug: **Propoxyphene**

Food: Alcohol

Outcome: This can be a dangerous mix. It can result in excessive (and possibly dangerous) sedation and depression of the central nervous system (e.g., loss of coordination, impaired judgment, decreased performance skills and alertness, slowed reaction time, increased risk of falls).This interaction has been associated with an alarming number of fatalaties.

What to Do: Avoid this mix.

P-59

Drug: **Propoxyphene**

Food: Food in general

Outcome: Food increases the time that propoxyphene remains in the stomach, resulting in increased drug absorption.

What to Do: Eat a healthy diet while on therapy. Your doctor will recommend dietary changes if they are indicated. Notify your doctor, nurse or pharmacist if you experience unusual or uncomfortable side effects.

P-60

Drug: **Propoxyphene**

Food: Smoking

Outcome: Smoking stimulates the liver to metabolize propoxyphene more quickly than normal. This can result in decreased drug effectiveness.

What to Do: It is best to avoid tobacco products for general health reasons. Notify your doctor, nurse or pharmacist if your therapy does not seem to be working effectively. Do not attempt to make dosage adjustments without consulting with a health professional.

P-61

Drug: **Propranolol**

Food: Alcohol

Outcome: The outcome of this interaction is unpredictable. Short-term use of alcohol can interfere with normal excretion of propranolol, resulting in increased blood levels, activity and adverse effects. Long-term use of alcohol can result in increased blood pressure, thereby decreasing the effectiveness of blood pressure therapy.

What to Do: In general, it's always best to avoid alcohol use while taking medications. Discuss alcohol consumption with a health professional if you plan to drink while on therapy. Notify your doctor, nurse or pharmacist if your therapy does not seem to be working effectively or if unusual symptoms occur.

P-62

Drug: **Propranolol**

Food: Food in general

Outcome: Food actually increases absorption of the drug.

What to Do: Take the drug at the same time each day in order to minimize the impact of food on therapy. Your doctor will recommend dietary changes if they are indicated. Notify your doctor, nurse or pharmacist if you experience unusual or uncomfortable side effects.

P-63

Drug: **Propranolol**

Food: High-protein meals

Outcome: High-protein meals interfere with normal metabolism of the drug. This can result in increased levels of the drug in the blood and increased drug activity.

What to Do: Eat a healthy diet while on therapy. Your doctor will recommend dietary changes if they are indicated. Notify your doctor, nurse or pharmacist if you experience unusual or uncomfortable side effects.

P-64

Drug: **Propylthiouracil**

Food: Foods high in goitrogens (e.g., brussels sprouts, cabbage, carrots, cauliflower, kale, pears, peaches, rutabagas, soybeans, spinach, turnips).

Outcome: These foods can interfere with the normal activity of propylthiouracil.

What to Do: Nothing is indicated. Eat a healthy diet while on therapy. Your doctor will recommend dietary changes if they are indicated. Notify your doctor, nurse or pharmacist if you experience unusual symptoms or if your therapy does not seem to be working effectively.

P-65

Drug: **Pyrimethamine**

Food: Folic acid

Outcome: Pyrimethamine can interfere with the normal metabolism of folic acid, resulting in decreased levels of it in the blood and deficiency.

What to Do: Eat a healthy diet. Your doctor will recommend dietary changes or supplements if they are indicated. Notify your doctor, nurse or pharmacist if unusual symptoms occur (see Appendix 13).

P-66

Drug: **Pyrimethamine**

Food: Para-aminobenzoic acid (PABA)

Outcome: PABA can interfere with the normal activity of pyrimethamine.

What to Do: Eat a healthy diet while on therapy. Your doctor will recommend dietary changes if they are indicated. Notify your doctor, nurse or pharmacist if your therapy does not seem to be working.

Q-1

Drug: **Quinacrine**

Food: Foods that acidify the urine (see Appendix 4)

Outcome: The drug is excreted more quickly than normal in acid urine. This can result in lower levels of quinacrine in the blood and decreased drug effectiveness.

What to Do: Eat a healthy diet while on therapy. Your doctor will recommend dietary changes if they are indicated. Notify your doctor, nurse or pharmacist if your therapy does not seem to be working.

Q-2

Drug: **Quinacrine**

Food: Foods that produce alkaline urine (see Appendix 5)

Outcome: Quinacrine may not be excreted as quickly in alkaline urine. This can result in increased levels of the drug and drug activity (including adverse effects).

What to Do: Eat a healthy diet while on therapy. Your doctor will recommend dietary changes if they are indicated. Notify your doctor, nurse or pharmacist if unusual symptoms or uncomfortable side effects occur.

Q-3

Drug: **Quinapril**

Food: High-fat foods

Outcome: Interference with normal quinapril levels and activity are theoretically possible. However, the actual clinical significance is not known.

What to Do: It is probably best to take quinapril on an empty stomach (1 hour before or 2 hours after meals) unless instructed otherwise by your doctor, nurse or pharmacist.

Q-4

Drug: **Quinidine**

Food: Food in general

Outcome: Food can delay absorption of quinidine.

What to Do: Quinidine is usually taken with food in order to avoid stomach distress.

Q-5

Drug: **Quinidine**

Food: Foods that acidify the urine (see Appendix 4), vitamins

Outcome: Quinidine is excreted more quickly than normal in acid urine. This can result in decreased drug levels and effectiveness.

What to Do: Eat a balanced diet. Your doctor will recommend dietary changes if they are indicated. Notify your doctor, nurse or pharmacist if your therapy does not seem to be working.

Q-6

Drug: **Quinidine**

Food: Foods that produce alkaline urine (see Appendix 5)

Outcome: Quinidine may not be excreted as quickly in alkaline urine. This can result in increased drug levels and activity (including adverse effects).

What to Do: Eat a balanced diet. Your doctor will recommend dietary changes if they are indicated. Notify your doctor, nurse or pharmacist if unusual symptoms or uncomfortable side effects occur.

Q-7

Drug: **Quinine**

Food: Foods that acidify the urine (see Appendix 4)

Outcome: Quinine is excreted more quickly than normal in acid urine. This can result in decreased drug levels and effectiveness.

What to Do: Eat a balanced diet while on therapy. Your doctor will recommend dietary changes if they are indicated. Notify your doctor, nurse or pharmacist if your therapy does not seem to be working.

Q-8

Drug: **Quinine**

Food: Foods that produce alkaline urine (see Appendix 5)

Outcome: Quinine may not be excreted as quickly in alkaline urine. This can result in increased drug levels and activity (including adverse effects).

What to Do: Eat a healthy diet while on therapy. Your doctor will recommend dietary changes if they are indicated. Notify your doctor, nurse or pharmacist if unusual symptoms or uncomfortable side effects occur.

Q-9

Drug: **Quinolone Antibiotics**

Food: Calcium, magnesium

Outcome: These drugs and nutrients bind together, which can interfere with normal absorption of the drug; decreased drug effectiveness is possible.

What to Do: It is best to take these drugs on an empty stomach (1 hour before or 2 hours after eating).

R-1

Drug: **Ramipril**

Food: Food in general

Outcome: The rate, but not overall extent, of ramipril absorption is reduced by food.

What to Do: Ramipril can be taken without regard to meals.

R-2

Drug: **Rifabutin**

Food: High-fat foods

Outcome: High-fat foods interfere with normal absorption of rifabutin, although the total extent of absorption is not affected.

What to Do: Rifabutin can be taken with foods, such as applesauce.

R-3

Drug: **Rifampin**

Food: Food in general

Outcome: The majority of reports indicate that food can decrease absorption, drug levels and activity of rifampin. However, some reports indicate that decreased absorption is more likely to occur with smaller doses (e.g., 150 mg) than with high doses (e.g., 750 mg).

What to Do: It is best to take rifampin on an empty stomach (i.e., 1 hour before or 2 hours after eating). Notify your doctor, nurse or pharmacist if your therapy does not seem to be working.

S-1

Drug: **Salicylates**

Food: Folic acid

Outcome: Chronic use of salicylates can interfere with the normal activity of folic acid.

What to Do: Eat a balanced diet while on therapy. Your doctor will recommend dietary changes or supplements if they are indicated. Report any unusual symptoms to your doctor, nurse or pharmacist.

S-2

Drug: **Salicylates**

Food: Foods that acidify the urine (see Appendix 4)

Outcome: Salicylates are not excreted normally in acidic urine. This can result in increased drug levels and enhanced drug effects (including adverse drug effects).

What to Do: Eat a balanced diet. Your doctor will recommend dietary changes if they are indicated. Report any unusual symptoms to your doctor, nurse or pharmacist.

S-3

Drug: **Salicylates**

Food: Foods that produce alkaline urine (see Appendix 5)

Outcome: Increased drug excretion in alkaline urine.

What to Do: Eat a balanced diet. Your doctor will recommend

dietary changes if they are indicated. It is probably best to avoid excessive intake of these foods while on therapy. Notify your doctor, nurse or pharmacist if your therapy seems not to be working effectively.

S-4

Drug: **Salicylates**

Food: Iron

Outcome: Iron deficiency has been reported.

What to Do: Eat a balanced diet while on therapy. Your doctor will recommend dietary changes if they are indicated. Report any unusual symptoms (see Appendix 14) to your doctor, nurse or pharmacist.

S-5

Drug: **Salicylates**

Food: Vitamin C (ascorbic acid)

Outcome: Decreased vitamin levels are possible, although this is more likely to occur with long-term use of salicylates. Decreased drug excretion is also possible, which could increase the effects of the drug (including adverse effects).

What to Do: Eat a balanced diet. Your doctor will recommend dietary changes if they are indicated. It is probably best to avoid excessive intake of vitamins while on therapy. Notify your doctor, nurse or pharmacist if unusual symptoms (see Appendix 24) occur, or if your therapy does not seem to be working effectively.

S-6

Drug: **Saquinavir**

Food: Food in general

Outcome: Food increases the level in the blood and activity of saquinavir.

What to Do: Saquinavir should be taken within 2 hours of eating.

S-7

Drug: **Secobarbital**

Food: Alcohol

Outcome: This can be a dangerous mix. It can result in excessive (and possibly dangerous) sedation and depression of the central nervous system (e.g., loss of coordination, impaired judgment, decreased performance skills and alertness, slowed reaction time, increased risk of falls).

What to Do: Avoid this mix.

S-8

Drug: **Sedatives**

Food: Alcohol

Outcome: This can be a dangerous mix. It can result in excessive (and possibly dangerous) sedation and depression of the central nervous system (e.g., loss of coordination, impaired judgment, decreased performance skills and alertness, slowed reaction time, increased risk of falls).

What to Do: Avoid this mix.

S-9

Drug: **Selegiline**

Food: Caffeine

Outcome: Excessive caffeine intake might cause a potentially hazardous increase in blood pressure.

What to Do: It is probably best to limit caffeine intake. Follow closely any dietary recommendations from your physician. Report any unusual symptoms to your doctor, nurse or pharmacist.

S-10

Drug: **Selegiline**

Food: Cheese

Outcome: An MAOI reaction (see Appendix 10) has been reported in at least one patient who consumed cheese while taking this drug.

What to Do: It is probably best to avoid tyramine-containing foods (see Appendix 7), especially in large amounts. Report any unusual symptoms (see Appendix 10) to your doctor, nurse or pharmacist.

S-11

Drug: **Senna**

Food: Calcium, fat, potassium

Outcome: Laxatives can interfere with the normal absorption of most nutrients. Nutrient deficiencies are possible, but are more likely to occur with chronic laxative use.

What to Do: The risk for nutrient deficiencies is small unless laxatives are being taken for long time periods. Report any unusual symptoms (see Appendices 12, 16) to your doctor, nurse or pharmacist.

S-12

Drug: **Serotonin Reuptake Inhibitors**

Food: Alcohol

Outcome: Impairment of mental and motor skills has not been demonstrated, but remains a concern among health professionals. Alcohol can increase the risk for problems in patients being treated for depression.

What to Do: Avoid this mix.

S-13

Drug: **Sertraline**

Food: Food in general

Outcome: Food increases the time required for sertraline to reach peak blood levels. However, higher than usual drug levels may eventually occur.

What to Do: It is probably best to take this drug on an empty stomach (1 hour before or 2 hours after eating).

S-14

Drug: **Simethicone**

Food: Ferrous (iron) sulfate

Outcome: Reduced iron levels in the blood have been reported.

What to Do: Simethicone is normally used only for short time periods. Eat a balanced diet. Report any unusual symptoms (see Appendix 14) to your doctor, nurse or pharmacist.

S-15

Drug: **Sleeping Pills**

Food: Alcohol

Outcome: This can be a dangerous mix. It can result in excessive (and possibly dangerous) sedation and depression of the central nervous system (e.g., loss of coordination, impaired judgment, decreased performance skills and alertness, slowed reaction time, increased risk of falls).

What to Do: Avoid this mix.

S-16

Drug: **Sodium Polystyrene Sulfonate**

Food: Sodium

Outcome: Increased sodium levels can occur.

What to Do: Sodium polystyrene sulfonate should be used with caution by patients on a sodium-restricted diet. Report any unusual symptoms (see Appendix 17) to your doctor, nurse or pharmacist.

S-17

Drug: **Sotalol**

Food: Food in general

Outcome: Reduced absorption of sotalol is possible.

What to Do: It is best to take this drug on an empty stomach (1 hour before or 2 hours after eating).

S-18

Drug: **Spironolactone (and other potassium-sparing diuretics)**

Food: Chloride

Outcome: Fluid and electrolyte disturbances are possible with any diuretics.

What to Do: Eat a balanced diet. Your doctor will recommend dietary changes if they are indicated. Report any unusual symptoms (see Appendices 16, 17) to your doctor, nurse or pharmacist.

S-19

Drug: **Spironalactone**

Food: Food in general

Outcome: Food causes the drug to remain in the stomach longer. This can increase absorption, levels of the drug in the blood and drug activity.

What to Do: Report any unusual symptoms or side effects of the drug to your doctor.

S-20

Drug: **Spironalactone**

Food: High-protein or high-fat diet

Outcome: Increased drug reabsorption has been reported.

What to Do: Eat a balanced diet. Report any unusual symptoms to your doctor, nurse or pharmacist.

S-21

Drug: **Spironolactone**

Food: High-fiber diets

Outcome: Increased excretion of spironolactone and possible decreased drug effectiveness can occur.

What to Do: Eat a balanced diet. Notify your doctor, nurse or pharmacist if your therapy does not seem to be working effectively.

S-22

Drug: **Spironolactone (and other potassium-sparing diuretics)**

Food: Potassium

Outcome: Increased potassium levels can occur.

What to Do: Eat a balanced diet. Avoid excessive potassium intake. Your doctor will recommend dietary changes if they are indicated. Report any unusual symptoms (see Appendix 16) to your doctor, nurse or pharmacist.

S-23

Drug: **Spironolactone (and other potassium-sparing diuretics)**

Food: Sodium

Outcome: Increased excretion of sodium has been reported. Fluid and electrolyte disturbances can occur with any diuretic therapy.

What to Do: Eat a balanced diet. Your doctor will recommend dietary changes if they are indicated. Report any unusual symptoms (see Appendix 17) to your doctor, nurse or pharmacist.

S-24

Drug: **Stavudine**

Food: Food in general

Outcome: Food can reduce stavudine levels in the blood. However, this does not appear to have a negative effect on therapy.

What to Do: Take the drug at the same time each day in order to reduce the impact that food might have on therapy. Notify your doctor, nurse or pharmacist if your therapy does not seem to be working effectively.

S-25

Drug: **Steroids**

Food: Calcium

Outcome: Decreased absorption of calcium can result in calcium deficiency and osteoporosis.

What to Do: Eat a balanced diet. Your doctor will recommend dietary changes if they are indicated. The use of illegal steroids (e.g., by athletes) is extremely hazardous to health. Report any unusual symptoms to your doctor, nurse or pharmacist.

S-26

Drug: **Steroids**

Food: Food in general (especially if high in fats)

Outcome: Increased absorption of the drug has been reported.

What to Do: Eat a balanced diet. Your doctor will recommend dietary changes if they are indicated. Report any unusual symptoms to your doctor, nurse or pharmacist.

S-27

Drug: **Steroids**

Food: Sodium

Outcome: Changes in normal sodium excretion can result in either increased or decreased sodium levels and activity.

What to Do: Eat a balanced diet and monitor weight gain (especially if due to water retention). Your doctor will recommend dietary changes if they are indicated. Report unusual weight changes or other symptoms to your doctor (see Appendix 17).

S-28

Drug: **Steroids**

Food: Vitamin A, zinc

Outcome: Decreased absorption of these nutrients is possible; deficiencies could occur over time.

What to Do: Eat a balanced diet. Your doctor will recommend dietary changes if they are indicated. Report unusual symptoms (see Appendix 18, 28) to your doctor.

S-29

Drug: **Streptomycin**

Food: Foods that produce alkalinize urine (see Appendix 5)

Outcome: Streptomycin is excreted more quickly than normal in alkaline urine. Alkaline urine enhances antimicrobial activity of the drug.

What to Do: Eat a balanced diet. This interaction is unlikely unless large quantities of these foods are consumed. Your doctor will recommend dietary changes if they are indicated. Notify your doctor, nurse or pharmacist if your therapy does not seem to be working effectively.

S-30

Drug: **Streptomycin**

Food: Foods that acidify the urine (see Appendix 4)

Outcome: Streptomycin is not excreted as quickly as normal in acid urine. This could result in higher levels of the drug in the blood and increased drug activity (including adverse effects).

What to Do: Eat a balanced diet. This interaction is unlikely unless large amounts of these foods are consumed. Your doctor will recommend dietary changes if they are indicated. Report unusual side effects or unusual symptoms to your doctor, nurse or pharmacist.

S-31

Drug: **Sucralfate**

Food: Food in general

Outcome: Food can interfere with the normal ulcer-binding effects of sucralfate.

What to Do: Take on an empty stomach (i.e., 1 hour before or 2 hours after eating). Notify your doctor, nurse or pharmacist if your therapy does not seem to be working.

S-32

Drug: **Sulfa Drugs**

Food: Food in general

Outcome: Food can interfere with the normal absorption of these drugs from the stomach and intestines. This can increase the time required for peak drug levels to be achieved.

What to Do: Take on an empty stomach (i.e., 1 hour before or 2 hours after eating) with a full glass of water. Notify your doctor, nurse or pharmacist if your therapy does not seem to be working.

S-33

Drug: **Sulfa Drugs**

Food: Alcohol

Outcome: Stomach irritation and nausea can occur.

What to Do: It is always best to avoid alcohol while taking any medications.

S-34

Drug: **Sulfa Drugs**

Food: Foods that acidify the urine (see Appendix 4)

Outcome: The drug is not excreted normally in acidic urine. This could result in increased levels and activity of these drugs (including adverse effects).

What to Do: Eat a balanced diet while on therapy. This interaction is unlikely unless large amounts of these foods are consumed. Your doctor will recommend dietary changes if they are indicated. Notify your doctor, nurse or pharmacist if your therapy seems not to be working effectively.

S-35

Drug: **Sulfadiazine**

Food: Food in general

Outcome: Food can interfere with the normal absorption of sulfadiazine from the stomach and intestines. This can increase the time required for peak drug levels to be achieved.

What to Do: Take on an empty stomach (i.e., 1 hour before or 2 hours after eating) with a full glass of water. Notify your doctor, nurse or pharmacist if your therapy does not seem to be working.

S-36

Drug: **Sulfasalazine**

Food: Folic acid

Outcome: Sulfasalazine can interfere with normal absorption of folic acid from the intestines. Over time this could result in a deficiency.

What to Do: Eat a balanced diet. Your doctor will recommend

dietary changes if they are indicated. Report unusual side effects or symptoms (see Appendix 13) to your doctor, nurse or pharmacist.

S-37

Drug: **Sulfathiazole**

Food: Foods that acidify the urine (see Appendix 4)

Outcome: Sulfathiazole is not excreted normally in acid urine. This can result in increased drug levels and activity (including adverse effects).

What to Do: Eat a balanced diet. This interaction is unlikely to occur unless large amounts of these foods are consumed. Your doctor will recommend dietary changes if they are indicated. Report unusual side effects or symptoms to your doctor, nurse or pharmacist.

S-38

Drug: **Sulfinpyrazone**

Food: Niacin

Outcome: It has been resported that niacin can interfere with some effects of sulfinpyrazone.

What to Do: Eat a balanced diet. Your doctor will recommend dietary changes if they are indicated. Notify your doctor, nurse or pharmacist if your therapy does not seem to be working effectively.

S-39

Drug: **Sulfisoxazole**

Food: Food in general

Outcome: Food interferes with normal absorption of sulfisoxazole. This can result in an increase in the time required for effective drug levels to occur in the blood.

What to Do: It is always best to take antibiotics on an empty stomach (i.e., 1 hour before or 2 hours after eating). If stomach distress occurs, contact your doctor, nurse or pharmacist for advice.

S-40

Drug: **Sulfonamides**

Food: Amino acids

Outcome: Sulfonamides can interfere with amino acid activity and protein synthesis.

What to Do: Eat a balanced diet. This interaction is unlikely to be a problem, since antibiotic therapy usually lasts for a few weeks or less. Your doctor will recommend dietary changes if they are indicated.

S-41

Drug: **Sulfonamides**

Food: Calcium

Outcome: Decreased calcium absorption can occur.

What to Do: Eat a healthy diet. This interaction is unlikely to be a problem, since antibiotic therapy usually lasts for only a few weeks or less. Your doctor will recommend dietary changes if they are indicated. Report unusual side effects or symptoms (see Appendix 12) to your doctor, nurse or pharmacist.

S-42

Drug: **Sulfonamides**

Food: Folic acid

Outcome: Decreased folic acid activity has been reported.

What to Do: Eat a healthy diet. This interaction is unlikely to be a problem, since antibiotic therapy usually lasts for only a few weeks or less. Your doctor will recommend dietary changes if they are indicated. Report unusual side effects or symptoms (see Appendix 13) to your doctor, nurse or pharmacist.

S-43

Drug: **Sulfonamides**

Food: Food in general

Outcome: Food interferes with the normal absorption of these drugs from the stomach and intestines. However, this is not necessarily a problem with all drugs in this category.

What to Do: It is best to take antibiotics on an empty stomach (i.e., 1 hour before or 2 hours after eating). If stomach distress occurs, notify your doctor, nurse or pharmacist.

S-44

Drug: **Sulfonamides**

Food: Foods that acidify the urine (see Appendix 4)

Outcome: These drugs are not excreted normally in acid urine. This can result in increased drug activity (including adverse drug effects).

What to Do: Eat a balanced diet and drink ample water. This interaction is unlikely unless large amounts of these foods are being consumed. Your doctor will recommend dietary changes if they are indicated. Report unusual side effects or symptoms to your doctor, nurse or pharmacist.

S-45

Drug: **Sulfonamides**

Food: Foods that produce alkaline urine (see Appendix 5)

Outcome: These drugs are excreted more quickly than normal in alkaline urine. This could reduce drug effectiveness.

What to Do: Eat a balanced diet and drink ample fluids (especially water). This interaction is unlikely unless large amounts of these foods are being consumed.Your doctor, nurse or pharmacist will recommend dietary changes if they are indicated.

S-46

Drug: **Sulfonamides**

Food: Magnesium, vitamin B_{12}

Outcome: Decreased absorption of these nutrients has been reported.

What to Do: Eat a balanced diet. Antibiotics are usually prescribed for only a few weeks. Thus, this interaction is unlikely to occur. Notify your doctor, nurse or pharmacist if unusual symptoms (see Appendix 15, 23) occur.

S-47

Drug: **Sulfonamides**

Food: Vitamin B_6 (pyridoxine)

Outcome: Inactivation of the vitamin can occur.

What to Do: Eat a balanced diet. Antibiotics are usually prescribed for only a few weeks. Thus, this intereaction is unlikely to occur. Notify your doctor, nurse or pharmacist if unusual symptoms (see Appendix 22) occur.

S-48

Drug: **Sulfonamides**

Food: Vitamin C (ascorbic acid)

Outcome: Crystal formation in the urine has been reported. If this occurs, it can result in kidney pain, painful urination, blood in the urine and kidney stone formation. Increased excretion and decreased activity of sulfonamides have also been reported.

What to Do: This problem is unlikely to occur except with a high intake of vitamin C, so, it is best to avoid excessive intake of the vitamin (more than 1 gram daily), especially while on therapy. Eat a balanced diet and consume ample fluids, especially water. Notify your doctor, nurse or pharmacist if unusual symptoms occur or if your therapy does not seem to be working effectively.

S-49

Drug: **Sulfonamides**

Food: Vitamin K

Outcome: Sulfonamide therapy can interfere with the normal production of vitamin K by the body. This could result in a vitamin deficiency with long-term therapy.

What to Do: This interaction is unlikely to occur because antibiotic therapy is usually prescribed for 2 weeks or less. Eat a balanced diet and drink ample fluds, especially water. Report any unusual symptoms (see Appendix 27) to your doctor, nurse or pharmacist.

S-50

Drug: **Sulfonylureas**

Food: Red wine and other alcoholic products

Outcome: It has been reported that sulfonylureas may interfere with normal alcohol metabolism. This could result in alcohol poisoning (e.g., flushing, nausea).

What to Do: Avoid this mix.

S-51

Drug: **Sumatriptan (oral)**

Food: Food in general

Outcome: Food can delay the time required for sumatriptan to work.

What to Do: Sumatriptan can be taken with food, although it may work more quickly when taken on an empty stomach (i.e., 1 hour before or 2 hours after eating).

S-52

Drug: **Surfactants (stool softeners)**

Food: Cholesterol, vitamin A

Outcome: Increased absorption and blood levels of these nutrients can occur.

What to Do: No interventions are necessary, especially with short term or occasional therapy with this drug. Your doctor, nurse or pharmacist will recommend dietary changes if they are indicated. Report any unusual symptoms (see Appendix 18) to a health professional.

S-53

Drug: **Sympathomimetics (e.g., nasal decongestants, some diet medications)**

Food: Foods high in pressor amines (see Appendix 7); tyramine, tyrosine

Outcome: It is theoretically possible for these nutrients to interfere with the normal metabolism of these drugs. This could result in a tyramine reaction (see Appendix 10).

What to Do: The actual risk of this interaction is very low. Eat a balanced diet and report any unusual symptoms to your doctor, nurse or pharmacist.

T-1

Drug: **Tacrine**

Food: Food in general

Outcome: Reduced drug levels and activity of tacrine have been reported.

What to Do: It is best to take this drug on an empty stomach (1 hour before or 2 hours after eating). However, it may be taken with food to avoid stomach distress.

T-2

Drug: **Terfenadine**

Food: Grapefruit juice

Outcome: Increased terfenadine blood levels can occur. This can result in increased activity (including adverse effects).

What to Do: It is best to take medications with water, rather than other beverages. Report any unusual symptoms to your doctor, nurse or pharmacist.

T-3

Drug: **Tetracycline**

Food: Aluminum, calcium, cheese, copper, dairy products, iron, magnesium, milk, mineral supplements, red meats, vegetables (dark green), zinc

Outcome: These nutrients form an insoluble complex with tetracycline and prevent it from being absorbed normally from the stomach and intestines. This can reduce the effectiveness of therapy.

What to Do: Take tetracyclines on an empty stomach (1 hour before or 2 hours after eating). Take with water.

T-4

Drug: **Tetracycline**

Food: Amino acids

Outcome: Interference with normal amino acid functions in the body have been reported.

What to Do: Antibiotic therapy is usually prescribed for 2 weeks or less, so this interaction is unlikely. Eat a balanced diet. Report any unusual symptoms to your doctor, nurse or pharmacist.

T-5

Drug: **Tetracycline**

Food: Folic acid

Outcome: Interference with normal folic acid functioning in the body and megaloblastic anemia have been reported.

What to Do: Antibiotic therapy is usually prescribed for 2 weeks or less. So, this interaction is unlikely. Eat a balanced diet. Report any unusual symptoms (see Appendix 13) to your doctor, nurse or pharmacist.

T-6

Drug: **Tetracycline**

Food: Food in general

Outcome: Food can interfere with the normal absorption of tetracycline. This can result in decreased drug effectiveness.

What to Do: It is always best to take antibiotics on an empty stomach (1 hour before or 2 hours after eating). Notify your doctor, nurse or pharmacist if your therapy does not seem to be working.

T-7

Drug: **Tetracycline**

Food: Potassium

Outcome: Tetracyclines can interfere with potassium utilization in the body.

What to Do: Antibiotic therapy is usually prescribed for 2 weeks or less. So, this interaction is unlikely. Eat a balanced diet. Report any unusual symptoms (see Appendix 16) to your doctor, nurse or pharmacist.

T-8

Drug: **Tetracycline**

Food: Vitamin A (high doses)

Outcome: Severe headaches have been reported. It is suggested that this occurs because of increased blood pressure in the brain.

What to Do: Avoid excessive intake of vitamin A while on therapy. Report headaches or other unusual symptoms to your doctor, nurse or pharmacist.

T-9

Drug: **Tetracycline**

Food: Vitamin B_2 (riboflavin), vitamin B_6 (pyridoxine), vitamin B_{12}, vitamin C (ascorbic acid), vitamin K

Outcome: Tetracyclines can inactivate some vitamins, interfere with their normal metabolism or production, or increase their excretion in the urine. With long-term therapy it is possible for a vitamin deficiencies to occur despite an appropriate diet.

What to Do: Eat a balanced diet. Discuss vitamin supplementation with your doctor, nurse or pharmacist if you will be taking the drug for more than a few weeks of therapy. Report any unusual symptoms (see Appendices 20, 22, 23, 24, 27).

T-10

Drug: **Theophylline**

Food: Caffeine, coffee, tea, cola beverages

Outcome: Caffeine can decrease the metabolism of theophylline by competing for the same metabolizing enzymes. Both caffeine and theophylline have stimulant activity (e.g., increased blood pressure, pulse, restlessness, upset stomach, nervousness, difficulty sleeping). Increased adverse effects can occur.

What to Do: It is best to reduce dietary intake of caffeine (less than 5-6 cups of coffee or tea daily), while on this therapy.

T-11

Drug: **Theophylline**

Food: Meat (barbecued, charcoal-broiled)

Outcome: These foods can increase metabolism and elimination of theophylline and interfere with drug effectiveness.

What to Do: It is best to avoid excessive intake of these foods. Notify your doctor, nurse or pharmacist if your therapy does not appear to be working effectively. Learn to use a peak flow meter to monitor therapy.

T-12

Drug: **Theophylline**

Food: Food in general

Outcome: Food can interfere with theophylline absorption and therapy.

What to Do: It is best to take theophylline on an emtpy stomach. However, it can be taken with food if it is irritating to the stomach. Talk with your doctor, nurse or pharmacist if therapy does not seem to be effective.

T-13

Drug: **Theophylline (Sustained Release; Long-Acting)**

Food: Food in general

Outcome: Food can increase the absorption and activity (including adverse effects) of some theophylline products (e.g., Theo-24).

What to Do: It is best to take long-acting products on an empty stomach unless you have been advised otherwise by your doctor, nurse or pharmacist.

T-14

Drug: **Theophylline**

Food: Cruciferous vegetables (large amounts)

Outcome: These foods can result in increased theophylline metabolism and interfere with the effectiveness of therapy.

What to Do: Avoid excessive intake of these foods. Eat a balanced diet. Notify your doctor, nurse or pharmacist if your therapy does not seem to be working effectively.

T-15

Drug: **Theophylline**

Food: Foods that acidify the urine (see Appendix 4)

Outcome: Theophylline is excreted more quickly than normal in acid urine. This can result in decreased levels of the drug in the blood and reduced effectiveness of therapy.

What to Do: Eat a balanced diet and drink plenty of fluids, especially water. This interaction is unlikely to occur unless large amounts of these foods are consumed. Notify your doctor, nurse or pharmacist if your therapy does not appear to be working effectively.

T-16

Drug: **Theophylline**

Food: Foods that produce alkaline urine (see Appendix 5)

Outcome: Theophylline is not excreted normally in alkaline urine. This can result in increased drug levels and activity (including adverse drug effects).

What to Do: Eat a balanced diet and drink ample fluids, especially water. This interaction is unlikely unless large amounts of these foods are eaten. Notify your doctor, nurse or pharmacist if you experience unusual symptoms or side effects.

T-17

Drug: **Theophylline**

Food: High-protein or low-carbohydrate diets

Outcome: These foods can increase metabolism and elimination of theophylline from the body. This can decrease drug activity and effectiveness.

What to Do: Eat a balanced diet and drink ample fluids, especially water. Your doctor will recommend dietary changes if they are indicated. Notify your doctor, nurse or pharmacist if your therapy does not seem to be working effectively.

T-18

Drug: **Theophylline**

Food: Low-protein, high-carbohydrate diets

Outcome: These foods can prevent theophylline from being eliminated normally by the body. As drug levels increase, adverse drug effects are more likely.

What to Do: Eat a balanced diet and drink ample fluids, especially water. Your doctor will recommend dietary changes if they are indicated. Report unusual side effects or symptoms to your doctor, nurse or pharmacist.

T-19

Drug: **Theophylline**

Food: Tobacco (nicotine), marijuana

Outcome: Nicotine increases normal metabolism and elimination of theophylline from the body. Thus, drug levels, activity and effectiveness are reduced. This interference can occur for up to 2 years after you have stopped using tobacco products.

What to Do: It is best to avoid tobacco products. If tobacco products are being used, monitor therapy carefully. Notify your doctor, nurse or pharmacist if your therapy does not seem to be working effectively. It is important to keep all physician and laboratory appointments in order to adequately monitor your therapy.

T-20

Drug: **Thiazides**

Food: Calcium

Outcome: Both decreased and increased calcium levels have been reported.

What to Do: Eat a balanced diet. Your doctor will recommend dietary changes if they are indicated. It is best to avoid calcium supplementation (especially excessive amounts) without first talking with a health professional. Report any unusual symptoms (see Appendix 12) to your doctor, nurse or pharmacist.

T-21

Drug: **Thiazides**

Food: Licorice (natural)

Outcome: Natural licorice can lower potassium levels, which in turn, can increase the risk for adverse effects due to these drugs. Natural licorice can also result in sodium and fluid retention, which would tend to increase blood pressure and work load on the heart.

What to Do: Avoid natural licorice when taking these drugs. Most contemporary candies and foods utilize artificial licorice flavoring, which is not a problem for therapy. However, natural licorice can be purchased from health and natural food stores. Always read product labels to see whether commercial products contain natural licorice or artificial flavoring. Report any unusual symptoms to your doctor, nurse or pharmacist.

T-22

Drug: **Thiazides**

Food: Magnesium

Outcome: Increased excretion of magnesium and significant magnesium losses can occur.

What to Do: Eat a balanced diet. Your doctor will recommend dietary changes if they are indicated. Report any unusual symptoms (see Appendix 15) to your doctor, nurse or pharmacist.

T-23

Drug: **Thiazides**

Food: Potassium

Outcome: Increased excretion and significant losses of potassium can occur.

What to Do: Eat a balanced diet. Talk with your doctor, nurse or pharmacist about increasing your dietary intake of potassium or taking potassium supplements. Report any unusual symptoms (see Appendix 16) to a health professional.

T-24

Drug: **Thiazides**

Food: Sodium

Outcome: Increased excretion and significant losses of sodium can occur.

What to Do: Eat a balanced diet. The average American diet contains as much as 10 times the amount of salt actually required by the body. Thus, sodium losses are often not a problem. Your physician will recommend dietary changes if they are indicated. Report any unusual symptoms (see Appendix 17) to your doctor, nurse or pharmacist.

T-25

Drug: **Thiazides**

Food: Vitamin D, calcium

Outcome: Increased levels and effects of vitamin D and calcium can occur (including adverse effects).

What to Do: Eat a balanced diet. Your doctor will recommend dietary changes if they are indicated. It is best to avoid supplementation (especially excessive amounts) without first consulting with a health professional. Report any unusual symptoms (see Appendices 12, 25) to your doctor, nurse or pharmacist.

T-26

Drug: **Thiazides**

Food: Zinc

Outcome: Substantial zinc loss can occur.

What to Do: Eat a balanced diet. Your physician will recommend dietary changes if they are indicated. Report any unusual symptoms (see Appendix 28) to your doctor, nurse or pharmacist.

T-27

Drug: **Thyroid, Thyroxine**

Food: Kale, cabbage, carrots, cauliflower, spinach, pears, peaches, brussels sprouts, turnips, soybeans, rutabagas.

Outcome: These foods can decrease thyroid hormone activity and interfere with therapy. Hypothyroidism can occur if these foods are taken in large quantities.

What to Do: Eat a balanced diet. It is best to avoid excessive intake of these foods. Notify your doctor, nurse or pharmacist if your therapy does not seem to be working.

T-28

Drug: **Ticlopidine**

Food: Food in general

Outcome: Increased levels and activity of ticlopidine can occur when it is taken after a meal.

What to Do: It is best to take this drug with food to avoid stomach distress. Take medications at the same time each day in order to make sure that your therapy is consistent.

T-29

Drug: **Tobramycin**

Food: Calcium, magnesium, potassium

Outcome: Losses of these nutrients can occur.

What to Do: Eat a balanced diet. Because this drug is normally used only for short-term therapy, nutritional supplements are not usually required. Report any unusual symptoms (see Appendices 12, 15, 16) to your doctor, nurse or pharmacist.

T-30

Drug: **Tolazamide, Tolbutamide**

Food: Alcohol

Outcome: Alcohol can result in unpredictable effects on sugar levels (increased or decreased) because of varied effects on drug metabolism. Additionally, the effects of alcohol on therapy can change over time. A disulfiram-type reaction (see Appendix 11) has been reported with some drugs of this type.

What to Do: It is best to avoid alcohol while taking this medication without first consulting your doctor, nurse or pharmacist.

T-31

Drug: **Tolmetin**

Food: Milk

Outcome: Decreased tolmetin levels have been reported, but this does not appear to have much effect on therapy.

What to Do: The drug is usually taken with food to avoid stomach distress. Take at the same time each day.

T-32

Drug: **Tolmetin**

Food: Food in general

Outcome: Decreased drug levels in the blood have been

reported, but this does not appear to significantly affect therapy.

What to Do: The drug is usually taken with food to avoid stomach distress. Take at the same time each day.

T-33

Drug: **Tranquilizers**

Food: Alcohol

Outcome: This can be a dangerous mix. It can result in excessive (and possibly dangerous) sedation and depression of the central nervous system (e.g., loss of coordination, impaired judgment, decreased performance skills and alertness, slowed reaction time, increased risk of falls).

What to Do: Avoid this mix.

T-34

Drug: **Triamterene**

Food: Folic acid

Outcome: It is thought that triamterene interferes with normal folic acid metabolism, especially with prolonged use. This can result in folic acid deficiency.

What to Do: Eat a balanced diet. Your physician will recommend dietary changes if they are indicated. Report any unusual symptoms (see Appendix 13) to your doctor, nurse or pharmacist.

T-35

Drug: **Triamterene**

Food: Potassium; potassium-rich foods (see Appendix 1)

Outcome: Increased potassium levels and adverse drug effects are possible.

What to Do: Eat a balanced diet. Your physician will recommend dietary changes if they are indicated. Report any unusual symptoms (see Appendix 16) to your doctor, nurse or pharmacist.

T-36

Drug: **Triazolam**

Food: Alcohol

Outcome: This can be a dangerous mix. It can result in excessive (and possibly dangerous) sedation and depression of the central nervous system (e.g., loss of coordination, impaired judgment, decreased performance skills and alertness, slowed reaction time, increased risk of falls). Fatal overdoses have been reported when this drug is taken with alcohol. This combination results in decreased elimination and higher blood levels of triazolam.

What to Do: Avoid this mix.

T-37

Drug: **Triazolam**

Food: Grapefruit juice

Outcome: Increased triazolam blood levels can occur. This can result in increased activity (including adverse effects).

What to Do: It is best to take medications with water, rather than other beverages. Report any unusual symptoms (e.g., increased sedation) to your doctor, nurse or pharmacist.

T-38

Drug: **Tricyclics**

Food: Foods that acidify the urine (see Appendix 4).

Outcome: In theory, these drugs are excreted more rapidly in acid urine, which could result in decreased drug activity. The risk of a significant impact on therapy is thought to be low.

What to Do: Eat a balanced diet and drink ample fluids, especially water (water tends to neutralize the urine). This interaction is unlikely to occur unless you consume excessive amounts of these foods. Your physician will recommend dietary changes if they are indicated.

T-39

Drug: **Tricyclics**

Food: Foods that produce alkaline urine (see Appendix 5)

Outcome: In theory, these drugs are not excreted normally in alkaline urine, which could result in increased drug activity (including adverse drug effects). Even so, the risk of a significant impact on therapy is thought to be low.

What to Do: Eat a balanced diet and drink ample fluids, especially water (water tends to neutralize the urine). This interaction is unlikely to occur unless you consume excessive amounts of these foods. Your physician will recommend dietary changes if they are indicated. Report unusual symptoms or side effects to your doctor, nurse or pharmacist.

T-40

Drug: **Trimethoprim**

Food: Folic acid

Outcome: Trimethoprim can block an enzyme that activates folic acid. This can interfere with folic acid metabolism and activity in the body, resulting in increased folic acid requirements and possibly deficiency.

What to Do: Eat a balanced diet. Your physician will recommend dietary changes or supplements if they are indicated. Report any unusual symptoms (see Appendix 13) to your doctor, nurse or pharmacist.

U-1

Drug: **Ulcer Medications**

Food: Alcohol

Outcome: Alcohol is irritating to the stomach, increases ulcer risk and interferes with ulcer healing.

What to Do: It is best to avoid alcohol while taking ulcer medications.

U-2

Drug: **Ulcer Medications**

Food: Caffeine

Outcome: Caffeine increases stomach acid production, increases ulcer risk and interferes with ulcer healing.

What to Do: It is best to reduce caffeine intake while taking ulcer medications.

V-1

Drug: **Valproic Acid**

Food: Alcohol

Outcome: This can be a dangerous mix. It can result in excessive (and possibly dangerous) sedation and depression of the central nervous system (e.g., loss of coordination, impaired judgment, decreased performance skills and alertness, slowed reaction time, increased risk of falls).

What to Do: Avoid this mix.

V-2

Drug: **Valproic Acid**

Food: Food in general

Outcome: Food can interfere with normal absorption of valproic acid, although this does not appear to be clinically significant.

What to Do: It is best to take valproic acid on an empty stomach. However, it can be taken with food in order to avoid stomach distress.

V-3

Drug: **Vasodilators**

Food: Sodium (salt)

Outcome: Salt interferes with the effectiveness of therapy.

What to Do: Eat a balanced diet. Your physician will recommend dietary changes if they are indicated. Even so, the average American diet contains as much as 10 times the amount of salt actually required by the body for normal functioning. Thus, lowering your salt intake is usually a healthy alternative. Using salt at the table, but not in cooking, offers a more healthy and tolerable alternative to our traditional dietary habits. Also, consider using lemon (it fools the tastebuds) on compatible foods as a salt substitute.

V-4

Drug: **Verapamil**

Food: Calcium

Outcome: Reduced drug effectiveness is possible. Verapamil works by interfering with the normal functions of calcium in the body. Calcium supplements or high calcium diets can interfere with therapy.

What to Do: Eat a balanced diet. Your doctor will recommend dietary changes or supplements if they are indicated. It is best to avoid supplementation (especially excessive amounts) without first consulting with a health professional. Notify your doctor, nurse or pharmacist if your therapy does not seem to be working.

V-5

Drug: **Verapamil**

Food: Grapefruit juice

Outcome: One study found that blood levels of verapamil were increased. This could result in increased activity (including adverse drug effects).

What to Do: It is best to take medications with water, rather than other fluids. Report any unusual side effects (e.g., slow pulse, constipation, lowered blood pressure) to your doctor, nurse or pharmacist.

V-6

Drug: **Verapamil**

Food: Iron, magnesium, zinc

Outcome: Verapamil binds with these nutrients and is not absorbed normally.

What to Do: Eat a balanced diet. Your doctor will recommend dietary changes if they are indicated. Notify your doctor, nurse or pharmacist if your therapy does not appear to be working effectively.

V-7

Drug: **Verapamil**

Food: Vitamin D

Outcome: Vitamin D increases calcium levels in the body. Verapamil works by interfering with the normal functions of calcium in the body. Calcium supplements or high-calcium diets can interfere with therapy. The therapeutic effectiveness of the drug may be reduced.

What to Do: Eat a balanced diet. Your doctor will recommend dietary changes if they are indicated. It is best to avoid supplementation (especially excessive amounts) without first consulting with a health professional. Notify your doctor, nurse or pharmacist if your therapy does not seem to be working effectively.

V-8

Drug: **Vinblastine / Bleomycin / Cisplatin Regimen**

Food: Retinol, vitamin B_1 (thiamine), vitamin B_6 (pyridoxine), vitamin E

Outcome: These drugs can decrease levels of these nutrients.

What to Do: Eat a balanced diet. Your physician will recommend dietary changes if they are indicated. Report any unusual symptoms (see Appendices 19, 22, 26).

V-9

Drug: **Vitamin A**

Food: Alcohol

Outcome: Alcohol interferes with vitamin A metabolism, which can result in increased vitamin levels. This can increase the risk for liver damage by alcohol.

What to Do: Avoid excessive alcohol or vitamin A intake.

V-10

Drug: **Vitamin A**

Food: Vitamin K

Outcome: Excessive intake of vitamin A can result in a deficiency of vitamin K.

What to Do: Avoid excessive intake of vitamins A and K without first talking with your doctor, nurse or pharmacist.

V-11

Drug: **Vitamin B_1 (Thiamine)**

Food: Alcohol

Outcome: Alcohol intake (especially chronic) can result in increased vitamin elimination and deficiencies.

What to Do: If you drink at all, do so only in moderation. Excessive alcohol intake results in numerous health problems.

V-12

Drug: **Vitamin B_1 (Thiamine)**

Food: Food in general

Outcome: Food can interfere with vitamin absorption, although this should not result in problems.

What to Do: Eat a balanced diet. Report any unusual symptoms (see Appendix 19) to your doctor, nurse or pharmacist.

V-13

Drug: **Vitamin B_1 (Thiamine)**

Food: Tannic acids (e.g., coffee, teas)

Outcome: Tannic acid binds with the vitamin and prevents it from being absorbed normally; vitamin deficiency is possible.

What to Do: Eat a balanced diet. Report any unusual symptoms (see Appendix 19) to your doctor, nurse or pharmacist. Take vitamins with water, rather than foods that contain tannic acids.

V-14

Drug: **Vitamin B_2 (Riboflavin)**

Food: Food in general, dietary fiber

Outcome: Increased vitamin absorption can occur; food increases the time that the vitamin remains in the stomach. This allows more time for the vitamin to be absorbed.

What to Do: No interventions are indicated. Eat a balanced diet.

V-15

Drug: **Vitamin B_{12}**

Food: Alcohol

Outcome: Alcohol can damage the mucosal lining of the intestines, which interferes with the normal absorption of the vitamin. Alcohol also interferes with normal vitamin metabolism. Decreased vitamin B_{12} levels and deficiency can occur.

What to Do: Eat a balanced diet. If you drink at all, do so only in moderation. Report any unusual symptoms (see Appendix 23) to your doctor, nurse or pharmacist.

V-16

Drug: **Vitamin C (Ascorbic Acid)**

Food: Foods that acidify the urine (see Appendix 4)

Outcome: Vitamin C is excreted more quickly than normal in acid urine. This can result in decreased levels and activity of vitamin C; vitamin deficiency is possible.

What to Do: Eat a balanced diet and drink ample fluids, especially water. This interaction is unlikely unless large amounts of these foods are consumed. Vitamin C deficiency is rare with normal diets. Report any unusual symptoms (see Appendix 24) to your doctor, nurse or pharmacist.

V-17

Drug: **Vitamin C (Ascorbic Acid)**

Food: Foods that produce alkaline urine (see Appendix 5)

Outcome: The drug is not excreted normally in alkaline urine. This can result in increased levels and activity.

What to Do: Eat a balanced diet and drink ample fluids, especially water. This interaction is unlikely unless large amounts of these foods are consumed. Report any unusual symptoms (see Appendix 24) to your doctor, nurse or pharmacist.

V-18

Drug: **Vitamin C (Ascorbic Acid)**

Food: Iron

Outcome: It is possible for iron levels to increase. Vitamin C can increase the capacity of the blood to contain iron. This is more likely to occur with a high intake of vitamin C and iron.

What to Do: Avoid excessive intake of vitamins and minerals. Report any unusual symptoms (see Appendix 14) to your doctor, nurse or pharmacist.

V-19

Drug: **Vitamin C (Ascorbic Acid)**

Food: Vitamin B_{12}

Outcome: Vitamin C has been reported to eliminate substantial amounts of vitamin B_{12}, resulting in deficiency.

What to Do: It is usually best to avoid excessive intake of vitamins (including vitamin C). Eat a balanced diet. Report any unusual symptoms (see Appendix 23) to your doctor, nurse or pharmacist.

V-20

Drug: **Vitamin D**

Food: Calcium

Outcome: Calcium levels may increase.

What to Do: Eat a balanced diet and avoid excessive intake of vitamins and minerals without first consulting with a health professional. Report unusual symptoms (see Appendices 12, 25) to your doctor, nurse or pharmacist.

V-21

Drug: **Vitamin A, Vitamin D, Vitamin E**

Food: Vitamin K

Outcome: Vitamin K deficiency can occur following excessive doses of fat-soluble vitamins.

What to Do: Avoid excessive intake of fat-soluble vitamins without first consulting with a health professional. Eat a balanced diet.

W-1

Drug: **Warfarin**

Food: Alcohol

Outcome: Chronic alcohol use can increase metabolism and elimination of warfarin and decrease its effectiveness. Light to moderate drinking does not usually affect the anticoagulant effects of the drug.

What to Do: It is best to avoid alcohol consumption, since alcohol might negatively affect therapy over time. If you drink, do so in moderation. Be sure to keep all laboratory and physician appointments so that your therapy can be effectively monitored.

W-2

Drug: **Warfarin**

Food: Broccoli, brussels sprouts, spinach, vegetables

Outcome: These foods can interfere with the normal activity of warfarin.

What to Do: Eat a balanced diet. Your doctor will recommend dietary and dosage adjustments if they are indicated. Keep all medical and laboratory appointments. Avoid fad diets and excessive intake of vitamins without first consulting with a health professional. Notify your doctor, nurse or pharmacist if your therapy does not seem to be working effectively or if you notice any unusual symptoms.

W-3

Drug: **Warfarin**

Food: Charcoal-broiled food

Outcome: Increased warfarin metabolism can occur due to increased activity of enzymes normally responsible for metabolism.

What to Do: Eat a balanced diet. Avoid excessive intake of these foods. Keep all medical and laboratory appointments. Your doctor will recommend dietary and dosage adjustments if they are indicated.

W-4

Drug: **Warfarin**

Food: Cooking oils with silicone additives

Outcome: Decreased absorption of warfarin can occur. Warfarin binds together with the silicone in the stomach and intestines and is not absorbed effectively.

What to Do: It's probably best to avoid these oils. Check the product label for ingredients. Keep all medical and laboratory appointments to insure that the drug is working effectively.

W-5

Drug: **Warfarin**

Food: Foods that acidify the urine (see Appendix 4)

Outcome: The drug is not excreted normally in acid urine. This could result in higher than expected levels of the drug in the blood and increased drug activity (including adverse effects).

What to Do: Eat a balanced diet. This interaction is unlikely to occur unless large amounts of these foods are consumed. Keep all medical and laboratory appointments. Your doctor will recommend dietary and dosage adjustments if they are indicated.

W-6

Drug: **Warfarin**

Food: Iron, magnesium, zinc

Outcome: These nutrients can bind with the drug and prevent it from working effectively.

What to Do: Take the drug 1 hour before or 2 hours after eating or taking vitamin/mineral supplements. Eat a balanced diet. Keep all medical and laboratory appointments in order to insure that the drug is working properly.

W-7

Drug: **Warfarin**

Food: Onions (boiled or fried)

Outcome: May increase some activities of warfarin.

What to Do: Eat a balanced diet. It is best to avoid excessive intake of onions while on therapy. Keep all medical and laboratory appointments. Your doctor will recommend dietary and dosage adjustments if they are indicated. Report any unusual symptoms or side effects to your doctor, nurse or pharmacist.

W-8

Drug: **Warfarin**

Food: Soy meal, Japanese food (which is high in soy meal)

Outcome: Increased activity of warfarin (including adverse effects, such as easy bruising and increased blood loss in the feces) can occur. The exact active substance in the food is not known.

What to Do: Eat a balanced diet. It is best to avoid excessive intake of these foods. Keep all medical and laboratory appointments. Your doctor will recommend dietary and dosage adjustments if they are indicated. Report any unusual symptoms or side effects to your doctor, nurse or pharmacist.

W-9

Drug: **Warfarin**

Food: Vitamin C (ascorbic acid)

Outcome: Vitamin C interferes with the anticoagulant effects of warfarin.

What to Do: Eat a balanced diet. Keep all medical and laboratory appointments. Your doctor will recommend dietary and dosage adjustments if they are indicated. Avoid fad diets and excessive intake of vitamins. Notify your doctor, nurse or pharmacist if your therapy does not seem to be working.

W-10

Drug: **Warfarin**

Food: Vitamin E

Outcome: The literature indicates that vitamin E can enhance the anticoagulant effects of the drug (i.e., increasing the possibility of hemorrhage), or that the combination may "undermine" the anticoagulant effects of the drug.

What to Do: Eat a balanced diet. Keep all medical and laboratory appointments. Your doctor will recommend dietary and dosage adjustments if they are indicated. Avoid fad diets and excessive intake of vitamins. Contact your doctor, nurse or pharmacist if you experience unusual symptoms.

W-11

Drug: **Warfarin**

Food: Vitamin K; foods which contain vitamin K

Outcome: Vitamin K can interefere with the ability of the drug to work effectively.

What to Do: Eat a balanced diet. Keep all medical and laboratory appointments. Your doctor will recommend dietary and dosage adjustments if they are indicated. Avoid fad diets and excessive intake of vitamins. Notify your doctor, nurse or pharmacist if you experience any unusual symptoms or if your therapy does not seem to be working.

Z-1

Drug: **Zafirlukast**

Food: Food in general

Outcome: Food can decrease absorption of zafirlukast by as much as 40%.

What to Do: Take zafirlukast on an empty stomach (1 hour before or 2 hours after meals).

Z-2

Drug: **Zalcitabine**

Food: Food in general

Outcome: Food interferes with normal absorption of zalcitabine and increases the time required to reach peak levels.

What to Do: Take as directed at the same time each day in order to avoid any impact which food might have on therapy. Notify your doctor, nurse or pharmacist if your therapy does not seem to be working.

Z-3

Drug: **Zidovudine (AZT)**

Food: Food in general

Outcome: Food decreases peak blood levels, but does not appear to affect overall therapy.

What to Do: Take as directed at the same time each day in order to avoid any impact that food might have on therapy.

Notify your doctor, nurse or pharmacist if your therapy does not seem to be working effectively.

Z-4

Drug: **Zinc (high doses)**

Food: HDL cholesterol

Outcome: Higher doses (e.g., 160 mg/day) can decrease HDL cholesterol levels. HDL cholesterol is the "good" cholesterol that helps to prevent heart problems. Thus, high zinc intake could theoretically increase your risk for coronary artery disease.

What to Do: Eat a balanced diet. Keep all medical and laboratory appointments. Your doctor will recommend dietary and dosage adjustments if they are indicated.

Z-5

Drug: **Zolpidem**

Food: Food in general

Outcome: Food interferes with normal absorption of zolpidem and might delay its activity.

What to Do: It is best to take the drug on an empty stomach (1 hour before meals or 2 hours after).

Z-6

Drug: **Zinc**

Food: Bran, brown bread, proteins, minerals (some)

Outcome: Decreased zinc absorption can occur.

What to Do: Eat a balanced diet. Your doctor will recommend dietary changes if they are indicated. Report any unusual symptoms (see Appendix 28) to your doctor, nurse or pharmacist.

Appendix 1

Nutrient content of selected foods (in milligrams per 100 grams).

FOOD	Sodium	Potassium	Calcium	Magnesium	Manganese	Iron	Copper	Potassium	Sulfur	Chloride
almonds	3	690	234	252	1.9	4.7	0.14	504	150	2
apples	1	116	7	5	0.07	0.3	0.08	10	5	4
apricots	0.6	440	17	9	0.2	0.5	0.12	23	6	2
artichokes	43	430	51		0.36	1.3	0.2	94	20	22
asparagus	2	240	22	20	0.19	1	0.14	62	46	53
avocados	3	340	10	30	4.2	0.6	0.4	42	25	10
bacon	1770	225	13	15		1.2		108		
bananas	1	420	8	31	0.64	0.7	0.2	28	12	125
beans (lima)	1	680	52	66		2.8	0.86	142	60	9
beans (string)	1.7	256	56	26	0.45	0.8	0.07	44	30	33
beef	65	355	12	24		3.2		196		
beets (peeled)	84	303	25	23	0.94	0.7	0.19	33	15	61
blackberries	4	181	32	24	0.59	1	0.12	19	17	15
bologna	1300	230	7			1.8		128		
bread (rye)	557	145	75	42	1.3	1.6	0.28	147		1025

Nutrient content of selected foods cont.

FOOD	Sodium	Potassium	Calcium	Magnesium	Manganese	Iron	Copper	Potassium	Sulfur	Chloride
bread (white)	507	105	84	22	0.31	2.5	0.2	97		
broccoli	15	400	103	24	0.15	1.1	1.4	78	137	76
brussels sprouts	12	450	29	20	0.27	1.5	0.1	80	78	40
butter (unsalted)	10	23	16	1	0.04	0.2	0.03	16	9	
buttermilk	57	147	109	16		0.1	0.02	95	30	100
cabbage	4	266	35	18	0.1	0.5	0.06	30		100
cantaloupes	12	230	14	17	0.04	0.4	0.04	16	11.7	41
carrots	50	311	37	21	0.25	0.7	0.08	36	21	40
cashew nuts	15	464	38	267		3.8		373		
cauliflower	16	400	25	7	0.17	1.1	0.14	56	29	30
caviar	2200	180	276			11.8		355		1800
celery	96	291	39	25	0.16	0.5	0.01	40	22	137
cheese (cheddar)	700	82	750	43		1		478		
cheese (parmesan)	755	153	1140	50		0.4	0.36	781	251	1110
cheese (swiss)	620	100	1180	55		0.9	0.13	860		1210
cherries	2	260	19	14	0.03	0.5	0.07	19	8	3
chicken	83	359	12	37	0.02	1.8	0.3	200		85
chives	3	250	76	32		0.9	0.11	26		

Nutrient content of selected foods cont.

FOOD	Sodium	Potassium	Calcium	Magnesium	Manganese	Iron	Copper	Potassium	Sulfur	Chloride
chocolate	19	397	63	107		1.4	1.1	142	32	
chocolate (milk)	86	420	228	58		1.1	1.1	251	67	151
clams	121	235	12	63		0.6		208		
coconuts	17	363	13	39	1.31	1.7	0.32	95	44	114
cod	86	339	11	28	0.01	0.5	0.5	190		97
coffee (unsweetened)	6	80	5	9	0.09	0.2		5		0.6
cod liver oil	0.1									
corn	0.4	300	3	38	0.15	0.7	0.06	111	32	14
corn oil										
cottonseed oil										
crab	1000	110	45	48		0.8	1.3	182		
cranberry sauce	1	17	6	2		0.2		4		
cucumbers	5	140	25	9	0.15	1.1	0.06	27	12	30
dates	1	790	59	65	0.15	3	0.21	63	65	290
egg (white)	192	148	9	11	0.04	0.2	0.03	17	208	161
egg (yolk)	50	123	141	16	0.09	7.2	0.02	569	194	142
eggplant	0.9	190	17	10	0.11	0.4	0.08	26	9	24
eggs (whole, raw)	135	138	54	13	0.05	2.3	0.03	205	197	159

Nutrient content of selected foods cont.

FOOD	Sodium	Potassium	Calcium	Magnesium	Manganese	Iron	Copper	Potassium	Sulfur	Chloride
figs	2	190	35	21		0.8	0.06	22	12	14
flounder	68	332	12	31	0.02	0.8	0.18	195		151
frankfurter	1100	230	7			1.9		133		
frog legs	55	308	18			1.5		147	163	40
garlic	32	515	38	36		1.4		134		
grapefruit	2	198	17	10	0.01	0.3	0.02	16	5	3
grapes	2	250	12	7	0.08	0.4	0.1	20	9	2
halibut	56	340	13		0.01	0.7	0.23	211		
ham (raw)	76	339	9	18	0.06	2.3	0.31	168		
ham (smoked)	2530	248	10	20		2.5		207		2060
hamburger (cooked)	47	450	11	21		3.2		194		
herring	118	317	57	26	0.02	1.1	0.3	240	202	122
herring (pickled)	1000		30	9				150		1600
herring (smoked)	720	285	66			1.4		254		23
0honey	7	51	5	3	0.03	0.5	0.2	6		29
horse radish	9	554	105	33		2	0.14	70	212	18
ketchup	1042	363	22	21		0.8		50		
lemons	6	148	26	9	0.04	0.6	0.26	16	8	4

Nutrient content of selected foods cont.

FOOD	Sodium	Potassium	Calcium	Magnesium	Manganese	Iron	Copper	Potassium	Sulfur	Chloride
lettuce	12	140	35	10	0.8	2	0.07	26	12	74
liver	116	292	7	15	0.27	6.5	2.1	352		
lobster	300	260	29	22	0.04	0.6	2.2	200	170	500
margarine (salted)	987	23	20					16		
mayonnaise	702	53	18	2		0.5		28		
milk (whole)	75	139	133	13	0.002	0.04	0.01	88	29	105
mushrooms	5	520	9	13	0.08	0.8	1.8	116	34	25
mustard (brown)	1307	130	124	48		1.8		134		
nectarines	6	294	4	13		0.5	0.06	24	10	5
olive oil	0.1		0.5			0.08	0.07			
olives (green)	2400	55	61	22	1	1.6	0.46	17	32	3750
onions	10	130	27	8	0.36	0.5	0.13	36	51	24
oranges	0.3	170	41	10	0.025	0.4	0.07	23	8	4
parsley	28	880	203	52	0.94	6.2	0.21	63	190	156
peaches	0.5	160	9	10	0.11	0.5	0.01	19	7	5
peanut butter	607	670	63	178		2		407	225	
peanut oil										
peanuts	3	740	74	181	1.51	2.2	0.27	407	377	7

Nutrient content of selected foods cont.

FOOD	Sodium	Potassium	Calcium	Magnesium	Manganese	Iron	Copper	Potassium	Sulfur	Chloride
pears	2	129	8	9	0.06	0.3	0.13	11	7	4
peas (green)	2	370	26	30	0.41	2	0.23	116	50	33
pecans		603	73	142	3.5	2.4		289		
perch	67	238	20			1		198		
pineapples	0.3	210	17	17	1.07	0.5	0.07	8	2.5	46
pistachio nuts		972	131	158		7.3		500		
plums	2	167	13	13	0.1	0.4	0.3	23	5	2
popcorn	3	240	11			2.7	0.31	281		
pork (chops)			11			3		235		
potato chips	340	880	40	48		1.8	0.36	139		
potatoes (raw)	3	410	14	27	0.17	0.8	0.16	53	29	35
potatoes (sweet)	5	530	32	31	0.52	0.7	0.15	47	15	85
prunes	6	700	51	32	0.18	3.9	0.16	79	28	9
pumpkins	1	457	21	12	0.04	0.8	0.08	44	10	37
radishes	15	260	30	15	0.05	1	0.13	31	37	37
raisins	31	725	62	42	0.32	3.5	0.2	101	42	9
raspberries	3	190	49	23	0.51	1	0.13	22	18	22
rice (whole)	9	150	32	119	1.7	1.6	0.36	221	121	

Nutrient content of selected foods cont.

FOOD	Sodium	Potassium	Calcium	Magnesium	Manganese	Iron	Copper	Potassium	Sulfur	Chloride
safflower oil										
salami	1260	302	35							2390
salmon (Atlantic)	48	391	29	29	0.01	0.8	0.2	266	190	64
sardines (drained)	823	590	437			2.9	0.04	499		
sauerkraut	650	140	36			0.5	0.1	18		
sausage (beef)	1130	255	21.2	16.6		4.1	0.17	168	163	1770
sausage (pork)	740	140	5			1.4		92		
scallops	150	420	26			1.8		208	342	
shrimp	140	258	63	42		2	0.43	300		
soybean oil										
spaghetti	5		22			1.5		165		
spinach	62	662	106	62	0.82	3.1	0.2	51	27	65
squash (summer)	1	202	28		0.14	0.4		29		
strawberries	1	145	21	12	0.06	1	0.13	21	12	11
sunflower oil										
tangerines	2	110	40	11	0.04	0.4	0.1	18	10	2
tea (unsweetened)	2	16	5	13	0.69	0.2		4		0.4
tomato juice	230	230	7	7		0.9		18		

Nutrient content of selected foods cont.

FOOD	Sodium	Potassium	Calcium	Magnesium	Manganese	Iron	Copper	Potassium	Sulfur	Chloride
tomatoes	3	268	13	11	0.19	0.6	0.1	27	11	51
trout	39	470	19		0.03	1	0.33	220		
turkey	66	315	8		0.03	1.5	0.2	212		123
turnips	37	230	39	7	0.04	0.5	0.07	30	22	41
veal	90	320	12			3		206		
vegetable oil	0	0	0	0	0	0	0	0	0	0
venison (round rump)	70	336	19	29		5		183	211	41
walnuts	4	450	99	134	1.8	3.1	0.31	380	146	23
water melon	0.3	100	7	8	0.02	0.5	0.07	10	9	8
yeast (baker's)	16	610	13	59		4.98		394		

Appendix 2

Vitamin content of selected foods (in milligrams per 100 grams unless stated otherwise).

FOOD	A (IU)	B_1	B_2	B_3	B_6	C	E	Folic Acid	K
almonds	75	0.25	0.92	3.5	0.1		15	0.045	
apples	90	0.04	0.02	0.1	0.03	5	0.3	0.002	
apricots	2700	0.03	0.05	0.7	0.07	7		0.003	
artichokes	160	0.08	0.05	1		9			
asparagus	900	0.18	0.2	1.5	0.14	33	2.5	0.11	
avocados	290	0.11	0.2	1.6	0.61	14		0.03	
bacon		0.36	0.11	1.8	0.35		0.4		
bananas	190	0.05	0.06	0.6	0.32	10	0.2	0.01	
beans (kidney)		0.6	0.22	2.1	0.28	2	4		
beans (lima)	290	0.24	0.12	1.4	0.55	29		0.13	
beans (string)	600	0.07	0.11	0.5	0.14	19	0.1	0.028	0.29
beef (loin, lean)	20	0.09	0.19	5.1					
beef (rib, lean)	20	0.09	0.18	5					
beef (round)		0.08	0.17	4.7	0.5			0.01	
beef (sirloin, lean)	10	0.09	0.19	5.2					

Vitamin content of selected foods cont.

FOOD	A (IU)	B_1	B_2	B_3	B_6	C	E	Folic Acid	K
beer		0.004	0.03	0.88	0.05				
beets	20	0.03	0.04	0.4	0.05	10		0.02	
blackberries	200	0.03	0.04	0.4	0.05	21		0.012	
brazil nuts	10	1	0.07	7.7	0.11	2	6.5	0.005	
bread (white)		0.25	0.21	2.4					
bread (whole meal)		0.3	0.1	2.8					
broccoli	2500	0.1	0.23	0.9	0.17	113		0.05	
brussels sprouts	550	0.1	0.16	0.9	0.16	100	1	0.05	3
butter	3300		0.01	0.1			2.4		
buttermilk (cultured)	35	0.04	0.18	0.1	0.04	1	0.05	0.0003	
cabbage (white)	70	0.05	0.04	0.32	0.11	46	0.7	0.08	
cantaloupes	3400	0.04	0.03	0.6	0.036	33		0.007	
carbonated drinks									
carrots	11000	0.06	0.06	0.6	0.12	10	0.45	0.008	
cashew nuts	100	0.43	0.25	1.8					
cauliflower	60	0.11	0.1	0.6	0.2	78	0.15	0.022	3.6
caviar									
celery	240	0.05	0.03	0.4		9	0.7		

Vitamin content of selected foods cont.

FOOD	A (IU)	B_1	B_2	B_3	B_6	C	E	Folic Acid	K
cheese (cheddar)	1310	0.03	0.46	0.1	0.07	10		0.016	
cheese (parmesan)	1060	0.02	0.73	0.2					
cheese (roquefort)	800	0.06	0.7	0.9					
cheese (swiss)	1140	0.05	0.33	0.1	0.09	0.5	0.35		
cherries	1000	0.05	0.06	0.3	0.05	10		0.006	
chicken (fryers)	170	0.1	0.2	6.8	0.5	2.5	0.21	0.003	
chocolate milk (sweet)	270	0.06	0.34	0.3			1.1		
clams		0.1	0.19	1.5	0.08			0.003	
coconuts		0.06	0.03	0.6	0.06	2	1	0.028	
cod		0.06	0.07	2.2	0.2	2		0.001	
cod-liver oil	85000						26		
coffee (unsweetened)		0.01	0.01	0.9					
corn (sweet)	400	0.15	0.12	1.7	0.22	12		0.03	
corn oil									
cottage cheese (creamed)	170	0.03	0.25	0.1					
cottonseed oil									

Vitamin content of selected foods cont.

FOOD	A (IU)	B_1	B_2	B_3	B_6	C	E	Folic Acid	K
crab		0.08	0.08	2.5	0.35			0.0003	
cranberries	40	0.03	0.02	0.1	0.06	12			
cucumbers	300	0.04	0.05	0.2	0.04	8		0.001	
dates	50	0.09	0.1	2.2	0.1			0.025	
egg (white, raw)		0.02	0.23	0.1	0.22			0.001	
egg (whole, raw)	1180	0.12	0.34	0.1	0.25		1	0.005	0.002
egg (yolk, raw)	3400	0.32	0.52	0.02	0.3		3	0.013	
eggplant	10	0.05	0.05	0.6	5				
figs	75	0.09	0.08	0.63	0.13	2		0.01	
flounder	30	0.22	0.21	3.8	0.25				
frankfurter		0.16	0.2	2.7					
frog legs		0.14	0.25	1.2		5			
grapefruit	80	0.04	0.02	0.2	0.02	40	0.25	0.003	
grapes	100	0.05	0.02	0.3	0.1	4		0.006	
haddock	60	0.06	0.17	3	0.2		0.6	0.001	
halibut	440	0.09	0.18	6	0.42			0.002	
ham (raw)		0.74	0.18	4	0.44			0.01	
hamburger (cooked)	40	0.09	0.21	5.4					

Vitamin content of selected foods cont.

FOOD	A (IU)	B_1	B_2	B_3	B_6	C	E	Folic Acid	K
hazelnuts	100	0.47	0.55	1.6	0.54	7.5	21	0.067	
herring	130	0.06	0.24	4.3	0.45	0.5	2		
honey			0.04	0.3	0.01	1		0.003	
ketchup	1400	0.09	0.07	1.6		15			
lamb (chop)		0.13	0.18	4.3	0.33		0.6	0.003	
lard									
lemons	20	0.04	0.02	0.1	0.06	45		0.007	
lentils (dried)	60	0.5	0.25	2	0.49		0.1		
lettuce	970	0.06	0.07	0.3	0.07	8	0.6	0.02	
liver (beef)	20000	0.3	2.9	13.6	0.7	31	1	0.29	
liver (chicken)	12100	0.4	2.5	10.8	0.8	35		0.38	
lobster		0.15	0.13	1.5		5		0.0005	
mackerel	450	0.15	0.35	7.7	0.7		1.6	0.001	
margarine (salted)	3300								
mayonnaise	280	0.02	0.04						
milk (breast)	330	0.01	0.04	0.18	0.02	5	0.23	0.0001	
milk (whole)	140	0.04	0.15	0.07	0.05	1	0.06	0.0001	
mushrooms		0.1	0.44	6.2	0.05	5	0.83	0.03	

Vitamin content of selected foods cont.

FOOD	A (IU)	B_1	B_2	B_3	B_6	C	E	Folic Acid	K
mustard (brown)									
nectarines	1650					13			
olive oil									
olives (green)	300	0.03	0.08	0.5	0.02			0.001	
onions	40	0.03	0.04	0.2	0.1	10	0.26	0.01	
oranges	200	0.1	0.03	0.2	0.03	50	0.23	0.005	
oysters	310	0.18	0.23	2.5	0.11			0.004	
parsley	8500	0.12	0.26	1.2	0.2	172		0.04	
peaches	880	0.02	0.05	1	0.02	7		0.004	
peanut butter		0.13	0.13	15.7	0.3			0.06	
peanuts	360	0.32	0.13	17.1	0.3		6.5	0.057	
pears	20	0.02	0.04	0.1	0.02	4		0.002	
peas (green)	640	0.32	0.15	2.5	0.18	27	0.6	0.025	0.3
pecans	130	0.86	0.13	0.9	0.19	2	1.5		
perch	30	0.075	0.12	1.7					
pineapples	70	0.08	0.03	0.2	0.08	17		0.004	
plums	250	0.07	0.04	0.5	0.05	6		0.002	
pork (loin, lean)		1.1	0.31	6.5					

Vitamin content of selected foods cont.

FOOD	A (IU)	B_1	B_2	B_3	B_6	C	E	Folic Acid	K
pork (ribs)		0.92	0.18	3.9	2				
potato chips		0.21	0.07	4.8		16			
potatoes (sweet)	8800	0.1	0.06	0.6	0.32	21	4	0.012	
potatoes (raw)		0.11	0.04	1.2	0.2	20	0.06	0.006	0.08
prunes	1600	0.1	0.17	1.6	0.5	3		0.005	
pumpkins	1600	0.05	0.11	0.6		9			
radishes	10	0.04	0.04	0.3	0.1	26		0.01	
raisins	20	0.11	0.08	0.5	0.3	1		0.01	
raspberries	150	0.03	0.09	0.9	0.09	25		0.005	
rhubarb	100	0.01	0.03	0.1	0.03	9	0.2	0.003	
rice (whole)		0.29	0.05	4.7			1.2		
rutabagas	580	0.07	0.07	1.1		43			
safflower oil									
salami		0.18	0.2	2.6			0.11		
salmon	220	0.17	0.17	7.5	0.98	1		0.002	
sardines (drained solids)	290	0.03	0.2	5.4	0.28				

Vitamin content of selected foods cont.

FOOD	A (IU)	B_1	B_2	B_3	B_6	C	E	Folic Acid	K
sauerkraut	50	0.03	0.04	0.2		14			
sausage (beef)									
sausage (bologna)		0.16	0.22	2.6					
shrimp	10	0.07	0.05	1.25	0.13				
spaghetti (unenriched)		0.09	0.06	2					
spinach	8100	0.1	0.2	0.6	0.2	51	2.5	0.075	3
squash	320	0.05	0.09	1		19			
strawberries	60	0.03	0.07	0.6	0.04	60		0.005	
sugar (brown)		0.01	0.03	0.2					
sugar (white)									
sunflower oil									
tangerines	420	0.07	0.02	0.2	0.07	31			
tea (unsweetened)			0.04	0.1		1			
tomatoes	900	0.06	0.04	0.6	0.1	23	0.27	0.008	
trout	150	0.09	0.25	3.5					
turkey		0.13	0.14	7.9				0.01	

Vitamin content of selected foods cont.

FOOD	A (IU)	B_1	B_2	B_3	B_6	C	E	Folic Acid	K
turnip greens	7600	0.21	0.39	0.8	0.98	139	2.3	0.04	
turnips		0.04	0.07	0.6	0.11	36	0.02	0.004	
venison		0.37	0.28	7.4					
walnuts	30	0.3	0.13	1	1	2	1.5	0.077	
watermelons	590	0.03	0.03	0.2	0.033	7		0.0006	
wine		0.005	0.01	0.05	0.09			0.001	
yogurt	145	0.045	0.024	0.18	0.05	2			

APPENDIX 3

Examples of Foods that Contain Selected Nutrients

FOLIC ACID

beans (navy)
cantaloupe
liver
nuts
oranges
vegetables (dark green, leafy)
whole wheat products
yeast

HISTAMINE

cheese (e.g., strong cheshire or swiss)
sardinella
skipjack
tuna (esp. spoiled)

PHOSPHORUS

cheese
egg yolk
liver
meat
milk
peanuts
whole grain cereals

POTASSIUM

almonds
apricots (dried)
artichoke
avocados
bananas
beans (kidney, lima)
beef
beets
brussels sprouts
cantaloupes
chestnuts (dried)
chicken (light meat)
coconut (dried)
corn (sweet)
dates
figs
fish (fresh)
garlic
grapefruit (fruit, juice)
hazelnuts
horseradish
lentils
liver (beef)
milk (dried, nonfat, whole)
mushroom
nuts (brazil)
onions (dried)
oranges (fruit, juice)

parsley
pea (dried, split)
peaches
peanuts (roasted)
pecans
pineapple juice
pistachios
pork
potato chips
potatoes (white, sweet)
prunes (fruit, juice)
raisins
sardines
soybeans
spinach
squash (winter)
tangerine juice
tomatoes
tomato juice and puree
turkey
veal
watermelon

SODIUM

asparagus (canned)
bacon
beans (canned)
buttermilk
caviar
cereals (most ready-to-eat brands)
cheese (processed)
crabmeat
crackers (salted)
frankfurters
mayonnaise
meats (canned)
meats (cold cuts)
olives (green)
pickles
potatoes (mashed)
pretzels
salmon (canned)
sardines (canned)
sauerkraut (canned)
tomato catsup
tomato puree (canned)
tuna (canned)
TV dinners

VITAMIN B_6 (PYRIDOXINE)

avocado
bacon
bananas
beans (kidney, lima, navy)
beef
bran products
cereal (whole grain)
fish
kidney (beef)
lentils
liver (beef)
meat (muscle, organ)
milk (whole, dry skim, malted)
molasses
oatmeal
peanuts
pork
potatoes
salmon (fresh)
soy beans
split peas
tuna
vegetables
walnuts
wheat germ
yams
yeast (baker's, brewer's)

VITAMIN K

- asparagus
- broccoli
- brussels sprouts
- cabbage
- cauliflower
- citrus fruits
- dairy products
- egg yolk
- fish
- fish oils
- fruits
- green peas
- green tea
- kale
- lettuce
- liver
- peas
- potatoes
- potato chips
- spinach
- turnip greens
- vegetable oil
- vegetables (leafy green)

APPENDIX 4

Foods that Acidify the Urine

bacon
brazil nuts
breads
cakes
cereals
cheeses
cookies
corn
crackers
cranberries
cranberry Juice
eggs
filberts
fish
fowl
grains
lentils
macaroni
meats
noodles
orange juice
peanut butter
peanuts
plums
poultry
prunes
rice
shellfish
spaghetti
vitamin C (ascorbic acid)
walnuts
whole wheat bread

APPENDIX 5

Foods that Alkalinize the Urine

almonds
beet greens
beets
buttermilk
chestnuts
citrus fruits
coconuts
crcam
dairy products
dandelion greens
fruits (except cranberries, prunes, plums)
kale
milk
molasses
mustard greens
nuts
spinach
turnip greens
vegetables (except corn and lentils)

APPENDIX 6

Foods Associated with the Development of Headaches

(see also APPENDIX 7)

aspartame
avocado
bananas
beans, lima
beans, navy
beans, pea
beans, pods of broad beans
bologna
breads (hot, fresh)
caffeine (excessive amounts)
cheese, brie
cheese, camembert
cheese, cheddar
cheese, emmentaler
cheese, gruyere
cheese, stilton
cheese, ripened
chocolate
citrus fruits
coffee (excessive amounts)
coffeecakes
donuts
fermented foods
figs, canned
foods with MSG (e.g., Chinese frozen dinners)
herring
hot dogs
liver, chicken
marinated foods
nuts
onions
peanut butter
pepperoni
pickled foods
pizza
pork
salami
sausage, fermented
sour cream
summer sausage
tea (excessive amounts)
vinegar (except white)
wines, red
yeast products
yogurt

APPENDIX 7

Foods that Contain Tyramine and other Pressor Amines

(see also APPENDIX 6)

avocado
bananas (large amounts)
bean curd
beer
bologna
bovril
broad bean pods
broad beans
caffeine (large amounts)
caviar
champagne
cheeses[1]
chocolate
figs, canned
fish[2]
ginseng
herring (pickled, spoiled, smoked)
liqueurs
liver (beef, chicken)
meat[3]
meat tenderizer
milk products[4]
miso soup
pepperoni
protein extracts
raisins
red plums
salami
sauerkraut
sausages (e.g., fermented, dry, summer)
shrimp paste
soups
sour cream
soy sauce
soya bean
spinach
teriyaki
tomatoes
whiskey
wine[5]
yeast extract

---

1 especially aged or strong, blue, boursault, brick (natural), brie, camembert, cheddar, emmentaler, gruyere, mozzarella, parmesan, processed, romano, Roquefort and stilton cheeses

2 especially dried and smoked; safer if fresh

3 especially game meats; fresh meats are safer

4 milk and yogurt appear to be safe

5 in general, but especially chianti, port, red, riesling, sauternes, sherry

APPENDIX 8

Physiologically and Pharmacologically Active Agents that Occur Naturally in Foods

ACTIVITY	FOOD EXAMPLES
allergy-causing	eggs, milk
antivitamins	soybeans (raw)
cancer or tumor-causing	apple cider, german raisins, yellow rice
cyanogenic glycosides	bitter almonds
depressants	lettuce (wild)
3,4-dihydroxyphenylalamine	beans
dopamine	(see Appendix 7)
enzyme inhibitors	legumes
estrogens	carrots, rice, wheat
favism-producing factors	beans (broad, fava)
goitrogens	rutabaga
hemagglutinins	castor bean
5-hydroxytryptamine	bananas, pineapple
hypoglycemic factors	akee fruit
metal-binding constituents	spinach
oxalates	spinach, rhubarb, celery
pressor amines, tyramine	(see Appendix 7)
salicylates	almonds, apples, apricots, blackberries, cherries, currants, gooseberries, grapes, raisins, wines, wine vinegar, nectarines, oranges, raspberries, strawberries
stimulants	coffee, tea, cola beverages

APPENDIX 9

Drugs Associated with Changes in Appetite

INCREASED APPETITE

- adrenal corticosteroids
- amitriptyline
- amoxapine
- anabolic steroids
- anti-inflammatory agents
- antipruritics
- benzodiazepines
- carbamazepine
- chlorpromazine
- cyproheptadine
- desipramine
- doxepin
- fluoxetine
- glucocorticoids
- haloperidol
- imipramine
- insulin
- lithium
- MAOIs
- maprotiline
- mesoridazine
- methysergide
- molindone
- nortriptyline
- oral contraceptives
- perphenazine
- phenothiazines
- psychotropics
- sulfonylureas
- thioridazine
- thiothixene
- tricyclic antidepressants
- trifluoperazine
- vitamin supplements

DECREASED APPETITE

alcohol
aluminum hydroxide (gel)
amebicides
amphetamines
anticonvulsants
antihypertensives
antineoplastics
benzodiazepines
biguanides
bulk-forming laxatives
carbonic anhydrase inhibitors
chloral hydrate
clofibrate
clonidine
colchicine
cytotoxic agents
digitalis
diuretics
estrogens
flurazepam
furosemide
griseofulvin
guanabenz
hydralazine
indomethacin
isoniazid
levodopa
lincomycin
lithium
MAOIs
methotrexate
methylcellulose
methyldopa
metronidazole
mineral oil
narcotics
penicillamine
penicillins (uncoated)
phenformin
phenothiazines
potassium-depleting diuretics
potassium-sparing diuretics
procainamide
pyrimethamine
spironolactone
stimulants
sulfasalazine
tetracyclines
thiazides
thiethylperazine
tolazemide
vitamin A
vitamin D

APPENDIX 10

Symptoms Associated with the "MAOI Reaction"

dangerous changes in blood pressure (high or low)
diarrhea
flushing
headache (severe)
itching
nausea/vomiting
palpitations (chest pounding)
stiff neck
sweating

APPENDIX 11

Symptoms Associated with the "Disulfiram Reaction"

- abdominal cramps
- blurred vision
- chest pain
- confusion
- dizziness
- flushing (e.g., facial)
- headache (throbbing)
- increased respiration
- light-headedness
- lowered blood pressure
- nausea/vomiting
- palpitations (heart pounding)
- shortness of breath
- sweating
- rapid pulse
- tears
- thirst
- throbbing in head and neck
- uneasiness
- weakness

SEVERE REACTIONS

- breathing difficulty
- convulsions
- death
- irregular pulse
- heart attack
- heart failure
- unconsciousness

APPENDIX 12

Calcium

Symptoms of DEFICIENCY:

- convulsions
- increased neuromuscular excitability
- muscle cramps
- numbness
- throat spasm

Symptoms of ADVERSE REACTIONS and EXCESSIVE Intake:

- abdominal pain
- anemia
- coma
- confusion
- constipation
- delirium
- depression
- diarrhea
- disorientation
- dizziness
- dry mouth
- frequent urination
- hallucinations
- impaired kidney function
- increased blood pressure
- increased urination frequency
- loss of appetite
- memory losses
- mental retardation
- nausea/vomiting
- ringing in the ears
- stupor
- thirst
- vague aches and stiffness
- weakness
- weight loss

APPENDIX 13

Folic Acid

Symptoms of DEFICIENCY:

- diarrhea
- forgetfulness
- inflammation of the mouth or tongue
- irritability
- low red blood cell count
- anemia (certain types)
- pallor
- shortness of breath
- sore mouth

Symptoms of ADVERSE REACTIONS and EXCESSIVE Intake:

- allergic reactions (rash, itching, difficulty breathing, malaise)
- confusion
- decreased vitamin B_{12} levels
- depression
- difficulty concentrating
- excitement
- impaired judgement
- irritability
- overactivity
- sleep disturbances

APPENDIX 14

Iron

Symptoms of DEFICIENCY:

anemia (various types)
a desire for strange foods (starches, dirt, ice)
belching
breathlessness
chronic nose disease with odorous discharge
constipation
decreased stomach acid
difficulty swallowing
dizziness
enlarged spleen
excessive menstrual flow
fatigue
gas (intestinal)
headache
heartburn
inflammation of the mouth and tongue
iron deficiency anemia
irritability
lassitude
loss of appetite
nausea/vomiting
nerve pain
numbness
palpitations (chest pounding)
shortness of breath (e.g., on exertion)
spooning of nails
stomach problems
swelling of the optic nerve
tingling
weakness

Symptoms of ADVERSE REACTIONS and EXCESSIVE Intake:

abdominal pain
black (blood-containing) stools
bleeding of stomach and intestines
blood clotting disorders
blood disorders
blood sugar changes (increased or decreased)
colon tumors
coma
confusion
constipation
cyanosis
decreased blood pressure
dehydration
diarrhea
disorientation
fluid swelling of the lungs
heart attacks
increased breathing frequency
increased susceptibility to infection
intestinal obstruction

- iron pigment deposits (skin, liver, pancreas)
- kidney failure
- lethargy
- liver failure or damage
- loss of appetite
- lowered blood pressure
- metabolic acidosis
- nausea/vomiting
- pallor
- pulse changes
- restlessness
- seizures
- shock
- stools may appear darker in color
- teeth stains

APPENDIX 15

Magnesium

Symptoms of DEFICIENCY:

- calcium deposits in the kidneys
- depression
- lowered calcium
- lowered potassium
- muscle spasms
- pulse changes (irregular, rapid)

Symptoms of ADVERSE REACTIONS and EXCESSIVE Intake:

- confusion
- changes in heart conduction
- difficulty urinating
- lowered blood pressure
- muscle weakness
- nausea/vomiting
- sedation
- skin warmth or redness
- slow pulse

APPENDIX 16

Potassium

Symptoms of DEFICIENCY:

- abnormal heart function
- changes in heart conductivity
- changes in urine composition
- confusion
- decreased reflexes
- depression
- drowsiness
- fatigue
- frequent urination at night
- intestinal obstruction
- irregular heart rhythm
- irritability
- lethargy
- malaise
- muscle cramps or spasms
- nausea/vomiting
- nerve damage
- numbness
- paralysis
- psychosis
- respiratory difficulty
- thirst
- weakness

Symptoms of ADVERSE REACTIONS and EXCESSIVE Intake:

- abdominal discomfort
- decreased reflexes
- diarrhea
- heart block
- changes in calcium levels (increased or decreased)
- irregular heart rhythm
- irregular heart conduction
- irritation of stomach or intestines
- kidney problems
- listlessness
- lowered blood pressure
- mental confusion
- muscle or respiratory paralysis
- muscle spasms
- muscle weakness
- nausea/vomiting
- numbness of extremities
- respiratory difficulty
- skin rash
- stomach / intestinal problems (obstruction, bleeding, ulcers, perforation)

APPENDIX 17

Sodium

Symptoms of DEFICIENCY:

- abdominal discomfort
- agitation
- apathy
- coma
- confusion
- decreased reflexes
- dccreased urine flow
- depression
- difficulty swallowing
- excitability
- gray skin
- hiccups
- intestinal blockage
- irritability
- lethargy
- loss of appetite
- muscle cramps, pain, spasm
- nausea/vomiting
- paralysis
- seizures
- somnolence
- stupor
- swelling (including brain, optic nerve)
- soft and sunken eyeballs
- vein distension
- weakness

Symptoms of ADVERSE REACTIONS and EXCESSIVE Intake:

- abdominal cramps
- coma
- convulsions
- diarrhea
- dizziness
- fluid accumulation in the lungs
- headache
- hypertension
- weakness
- fluid accumulation
- irritability
- muscular twitching
- nausea/vomiting
- rapid pulse
- respiratory arrest
- restlessness
- swelling

APPENDIX 18

Vitamin A

Symptoms of DEFICIENCY

birth defects
bone changes
death
decreased hormone production
difficulty walking
eye problems (irritation, damage, dryness)
general decline in health and growth
increased pressure of the brain
lowered resistance to infections
miscarriage
night blindness
skin changes (dry, flaking, scaly, rough)
thickening of bone

Symptoms of ADVERSE EFFECTS and EXCESSIVE Intake

abdominal discomfort
alopecia (hair loss)
anorexia (loss of appetite)
vision disturbances (blurred or double)
bone problems (breakdown, thickening, pain, tenderness)
brittle nails
cirrhosis of the liver
constipation
death
diarrhea
dizziness
drowsiness
dry mucous membranes (e.g., nose, throat)
enlarged spleen or liver
fatigue
fractures
frequent urination
headache
increased fluid pressure of brain or spine
increased skin pigmentation
increased thirst
inflammation of tongue, lips, gums
irritability
itching
jaundice
joint pain
lethargy
liver damage
malaise
menstrual changes
muscle soreness or stiffness
nausea/vomiting

night sweats
reddish pimples on shoulders and back
skeletal abnormalities
skin problems (dry, flaking, itching, redness, peeling, scaling, discoloration)
slow growth
swelling of legs or feet
thickening of skin and bones

APPENDIX 19

Vitamin B_1 (Thiamine)

Symptoms of DEFICIENCY:

Deficiency Disease: BERIBERI

- congestive heart failure
- constipation
- depression
- difficulty walking
- enlarged heart
- fatigue
- headache
- heart/blood vessel abnormalities
- heart failure
- insomnia
- irritability
- lack of initiative
- loss of appetite
- mental confusion
- muscle tenderness or weakness
- palpitations (chest or heart pounding)
- paralysis
- personality disturbances
- poor memory
- rapid pulse
- sensory disturbances in the extremities (increased or decreased)
- shortness of breath (esp. on exertion)
- stomach/intestinal problems
- swelling (e.g., legs)
- visual problems
- weakness

Symptoms of ADVERSE REACTIONS and EXCESSIVE Intake:

- bleeding of stomach or intestines
- cyanosis
- death
- feeling of warmth
- fluid accumulation in the lungs
- heart problems
- itching
- nausea/vomiting
- restlessness
- stomach/abdominal discomfort
- throat tightness
- sweating
- swelling
- weakness

APPENDIX 20

Vitamin B_2 (Riboflavin)

Symptoms of DEFICIENCY:

Deficiency Disease: ARIBOFLAVINOSIS

anemia
eyelid spasm (excessive winking)
blurred vision
burning, irritation, soreness (eyes, lips, tongue, mouth)
cracks at the corners of the mouth
skin irritation (e.g., on the face, trunk, extremities)
light-headedness
light sensitivity (intolerance)
itching eyes
nerve abnormalities
roughness of eyelids

Symptoms of ADVERSE REACTIONS and EXCESSIVE Intake:

bright yellow urine
diarrhea
nausea/vomiting
stomach pain

APPENDIX 21

Vitamin B_3 (Niacin, Nicotinic Acid)

Symptoms of DEFICIENCY:

Deficiency Disease: PELLAGRA

blood disorders
confusion
dementia
depression
dermatitis
diarrhea
dizziness
hallucinations
headache
inflammation of the stomach and intestines
insomnia
nausea/vomiting
poor memory
salivary gland changes (excessive secretions, swelling)
sunburn-like areas on the skin
tongue problems (sores, swelling, redness)

Symptoms of ADVERSE REACTIONS and EXCESSIVE Intake:

abdominal pain
abnormal blood sugar tolerance
abnormal liver function
activation of peptic ulcer
diarrhea
dizziness
feeling of warmth
flushing
irritation of stomach and intestines
headache
heartburn
increased intestinal activity
increased uric acid in the blood
irregular pulse
itching
liver damage
low blood pressure
nausea/vomiting
skin changes (dryness, pigmentation, growths, rash)
vascular changes

APPENDIX 22

Vitamin B_6 (Pyridoxine)

Symptoms of DEFICIENCY

abnormal EEG
anemia (certain types)
carpal tunnel syndrome[1]
CNS lesions
convulsions
depression
disorders of the nerves
inflammation or sores
(eyes, mouth, nose and tongue)
irritability
memory loss
seborrhea-like skin lesions
(face, eyes, nose, mouth)
seizures

Symptoms of ADVERSE REACTIONS and EXCESSIVE Intake:

abnormal EEG
awkwardness of hands
decreased sensation
(touch, temperature,
vibration)
disorders of the sensory
nerves
impaired memory
muscle incoordination
nervousness
numbness (feet, mouth)
sleepiness
tremors
unstable gait
Vitamin B_6 dependency
(transient, upon withdrawal)

---

1 However, even when carpal tunnel syndrome is related to B_6 deficiency, it does NOT appear that taking more vitamins will cure the problem.

APPENDIX 23

Vitamin B_{12} (Cyanocobalamin)

Symptoms of DEFICIENCY:

anemia (certain types)
cell abnormalities
(e.g., bone, blood)
changes in the stomach
and intestines
confusion
decreased reflexes
(deep tendon)
decreased sensory
perceptions (touch)
delusions or hallucinations
inflammation of the tongue
visual disturbances
memory losses
mood changes
nerve degeneration and damage
(can be permanent with
prolonged and
severe deficiency)
numbness (hands and feet)
psychiatric disturbances
unsteadiness

Symptoms of ADVERSE REACTIONS and EXCESSIVE Intake:

acne (rare)
allergy reactions
clots
congestive heart failure
fluid accumulation in the lungs
itching
skin eruptions

APPENDIX 24

Vitamin C (Ascorbic Acid)

Symptoms of DEFICIENCY:

Deficiency Disease: SCURVY

aching (joint, muscles)
anemia
bleeding
(gums, mouth, intestinal tract, skin surface, mucus membranes)
capillary fragility and bruising
degenerative changes
(capillaries, bone and connective tissues)
faulty bone and tooth development
gingivitis
gums problems (swollen, weak, spongy)
impaired wound healing
loose teeth
loss of appetite
prominent hair follicles
weakness

Symptoms of ADVERSE REACTIONS and EXCESSIVE Intake[1]:

can trigger diabetes
dental erosion (severe)[2]
kidney stones
(can precipitate certain types of stones, especially with high doses)
diarrhea
enhanced fertility
(via thinning of uterine mucus)
fainting or dizziness
(with rapid IV administration)
false laboratory tests
(blood, urine and stool)
"rebound scurvy" (after stopping chronic ingestion of large doses)
soreness at injection sites
(transient and mild)

---

1 serious toxicity is uncommon

2 was reported in a patient who took high daily doses for 3 years

APPENDIX 25

Vitamin D

Symptoms of DEFICIENCY

Deficiency Disease: RICKETS (in children)

bone pain (back, thighs, shoulders, ribs)
deformity
difficulty walking
growth arrest
hearing loss (progressive)
low calcium levels
low phosphorus levels
muscle weakness (e.g., legs)
osteomalacia (adults)

Symptoms of ADVERSE REACTIONS and EXCESSIVE Intake:

aches and stiffness (vague)
acidosis (mild)
anemia
bad taste in mouth (e.g., metallic)
bone mineralization (in children)
calcium deposits in soft tissues
cataracts
CNS changes
constipation
convulsions
death (due to failure of heart or kidneys)
decreased growth rate (in children)
decreased sex drive
diarrhea
dry mouth
excess calcium levels
excessive nitrogen in the blood or urine (reversible)
eye redness
fatigue
frequent urination at night
headache
heart abnormalities (in fetus)
increased blood pressure
increased calcium levels (blood and urine)
inflammation of the pancreas
irregular heart rhythms
irritability
itching
kidney problems
(decreased functioning, damage, stones)
liver damage
loss of appetite
malaise (loss of energy, feeling "sick")
mental retardation
nausea/vomiting
osteoporosis (loss of calcium from bones)

- pain (vague; muscle and bone)
- parathyroid suppression[1]
- runny nose
- sensitivity to light
- sleepiness
- thirst
- ulcers (peptic)
- urine abnormalities
- weakness
- weight loss

---

1 In neonates born to mothers with maternal hypervitaminosis.

APPENDIX 26

Vitamin E

Symptoms of DEFICIENCY:

anemia
decreased reflexes
loss of coordination
loss of vibratory sensation
muscle weakness
nerve disturbances
visual problems
(impaired acuity and night vision)

Symptoms of ADVERSE REACTIONS and EXCESSIVE Intake:

abdominal cramps
blurred vision
breast tenderness
diarrhea
elevated blood sugar levels
fatigue
gas (intestinal)
headache
hives or rash
increased blood pressure
muscle problems
nausea
weakness

APPENDIX 27

Vitamin K

Symptoms of DEFICIENCY:

- bleeding of stomach or intestines
- blood in the urine
- bruising
- decreased clotting ability
- increased tendency to bleed
- nosebleed

Symptoms of ADVERSE REACTIONS and EXCESSIVE Intake:

Phytonadione
- chest pain
- death (has occurred after IV administration)
- flushing
- hives, rash, itching
- shortness of breath
- skin rash

Menadione
- blood disorders
- enlarged spleen
- kidney damage
- liver damage

APPENDIX 28

Zinc

Symptoms of DEFICIENCY:

- decreased functioning of testes or ovaries
- disturbances of vision, smell, taste
- dwarfism
- enlargement of liver and spleen
- inflammation (eyelids, mouth, nails, tongue)
- hair loss
- impaired healing
- impaired taste
- loss of appetite
- rashes
- retarded growth
- skin lesions

Symptoms of ADVERSE REACTIONS and EXCESSIVE Intake:

- dehydration
- diarrhea
- drowsiness
- increased levels of some enzymes
- lethargy
- nausea/vomiting
- rash
- restlessness

APPENDIX 29

Drug Brand Name Conversion Chart

The food/drug interactions included in this book have been compiled using the generic name of the drug, or in some cases, by drug category. The following listing has been compiled alphabetically by example brand names to assist the reader in locating appropriate listings in the text. Health professionals will note that the salt form has not been included with the generic names in this listing for the sake of brevity and simplicity.

Brand Name	Generic Name(s)	Category
Accupril	quinapril	Blood Pressure: ACE Inhibitor
Accurbron	theophylline	Bronchodilator: Xanthine
Accutane	isotretinoin (retinoic acid)	Acne
Achromycin V	tetracycline	Antibiotic: Tetracycline
Adalat	nifedipine	Calcium Channel Blocker
Adapin	doxepin	Antidepressant: Tricyclic
Adipex-P	phentermine	Anorexiant: Amphetamine-like
Adrucil	5-fluorouracil (5-FU)	Cancer: Antimetabolite
Advil	ibuprofen	Analgesic: NSAID
AeroBid	flunisolide	Corticosteroid
Aerolate	theophylline	Bronchodilator: Xanthine
Aerosporin	polymyxin B	Antibiotic
Afrin	oxymetazoline	Decongestant
Agoral	mineral oil	Laxative: Emolient
Akineton	biperiden	Parkinsons: Anticholinergic
Albamycin	novobiocin	Antibiotic
Aldactazide	hydrochlorothizaide, spironolactone	Diuretic: Thiazide/Potassium Sparing
Aldactone	spironolactone	Diuretic: Potassium Sparing
Aldochlor	chlorothiazide, methyldopa	Blood Pressure: Diuretic/ Methyldopa
Aldomet	methyldopa	Blood Pressure: Methyldopa

Brand Name	Generic Name(s)	Category
Aldoril D	hydrochlorothiazide	Diuretic: Thiazide
Aleve	naproxen	Analgesic: NSAID
Alka Seltzer	sodium bicarbonate	Antacid
Altace	ramipril	High Blood Pressure: ACE Inhibitor
AlternaGEL	aluminum hydroxide	Antacid
Aludrox	aluminum hydroxide, magnesium hydroxide	Antacid
Alupent	metaproterenol	Asthma: Bronchodilator/ Sympathomimetic
Alurate	aprobarbital	Sedative: Barbiturate
Ambien	zolpidem	Sedative: Miscellaneous
Amen	medroxyprogesterone	Progestin
Amoxil	amoxicillin	Antibiotic: Penicillin
Amphojel	aluminum hydroxide	Antacid
Anadrol	oxymetholone	Anabolic Steroid
Anafranil	chlomipramine	Antidepressant: Tricyclic
Anaprox	naproxen	Analgesic: NSAID
Anaspaz	hyoscyamine	Ulcer/GI: Anticholinergic
Ancobon	flucytosine	Antifungal
Android	methyltestosterone	Androgen
Anexsia	hydrocodone, acetaminophen	Analgesic Combination: Narcotic/ Acetaminophen
Ansaid	flurbiprofen	Analgesic: NSAID
Antabuse	disulfiram	Alcohol Deterrent
Antivert	meclizine	Motion Sickness: Antihistamine
Anturane	sulfinpyrazone	Gout Agent
Apresazide	hydrochlorothiazide, hydralazine	High Blood Pressure: Thiazide/ Vasodilator
Apresoline	hydralazine	High Blood Pressure: Vasodilator
Aquatensen	methyclothiazide	Diuretic: Thiazide
Aralen	chloroquine	Malaria
Aristocort	triamcinolone	Adrenal Steroid: Glucocorticoid
Armour Thyroid	thyroid	Thyroid Hormone
Artane	trihexphenidyl	Parkinsons: Anticholinergic

Brand Name	Generic Name(s)	Category
Asbron G	theophylline, guaifenesin	Asthma: Xanthine Bronchodilator/Expectorant
Ascorbis Acid	vitamin C	Vitamin
Asendin	amoxapine	Antidepressant: Tricyclic
Atabrine	quinacrine	Antibiotic: Amebicide
Atarax	hydroxyzine	AntiAnxiety
Ativan	iorazepam	AntiAnxiety: Benzodiazepine
Atromid S	clofibrate	Cholesterol/Lipid Lowering Agent
Augmentin	amoxicillin, potassium clavulanate	Antiobiotic: Penicillin
Aureomycin	chlortetracycline	Antibiotic: Tetracycline
Aventyl	nortriptyline	Antidepressant: Tricyclic
Axid	nizatidine	H2 Blocker
Aygestin	norethindrone	Progestin
Azmacort	triamcinolone	Adrenal Steroid: Corticosteroid
Azo Gantrisin	sulfisoxazole, phenazopyridine	Antibiotic: Sulfa
Azulfidine	sulfasalazine	Antibiotic: Sulfa
Bactocill	oxacillin	Antibiotic: Penicillin
Bactrim	sulfamethoxazole trimethoprim	Antibiotic: Sulfa
Bancap HC	hydrocodone, acetaminophen	Analgesic: Narcotic/ Acetaminophen
Banthine	methantheline	Ulcer/GI: Anticholinergic
Beclovent	beclomethasone	Adrenal Steroid: Corticosteroid
Beepen-VK	penicillin V	Antibiotic: Penicillin
Bellergal-S	belladonna alkaloids, phenobarbital	Ulcer/GI: Anticholinergic/ Barbiturate
Benadryl	diphenhydramine	Anthihistamine
Benemid	probenecid	Gout
Bentyl	dicyclomine	Ulcer/GI: Anticholinergic
Benylin	diphenhydramine	Antihistamine
Beta-Carotene	provitamin A	Vitamin
Betapace	sotalol	Blood Pressure/Heart: Beta-Blocker

Brand Name	Generic Name(s)	Category
Biaxin	clarithromycin	Antibiotic: Macrolide
Bioflavonoids	vitamin P	Vitamin
Black-Draught	senna	Laxative: Stimulant
Blenoxane	bleomycin	Cancer: Antibiotic
Blocadren	timilol	Blood Pressure/Heart: Beta-Blocker
Bonine	meclizine	Motion Sickness: Antihistamine
Bontril PDM	phendimetrazine	Anorexiant: Amphetamine-like
Brethaire	terbutaline	Asthma: Bronchodilator/ Sympathomimetic
Brethine	terbutaline	Asthma: Bronchodilator/ Sympathomimetic
Brevibloc	esmolol	Blood Pressure/Heart: Beta-Blocker
Brevicon	ethinyl estradiol, ethynodial diacetate	Contraceptive (Oral): Estrogen/Progestin
Bricanyl	terbutaline	Asthma: Bronchodilator/ Sympathomimetic
Bronkaid Mist	epinephrine	Asthma: Bronchodilator/ Sympathomimetic
Bronkodyl	theophylline	Asthma: Bronchodilator/Xanthine
Bucladin-S	buclizine	Motion Sickness: Antihistamine
Bumex	bumetanide	Diuretic: Loop
BuSpar	buspirone	AntiAnxiety
Butazolidin	phenylbutazone	Analgesic: NSAID
Butisol	butabarbital	Sedative: Barbiturate
Cafergot	ergotamine, caffeine	Migraine
Calan	verapamil	Blood Pressure/Heart: Calcium Channel Blocker
Cantil	mepenzolate,	Ulcer/GI: Anticholinergic
Capoten	captopril	Blood Pressure: ACE Inhibitor
Capozide	hydrocholorthiazide, captopril	Blood Pressure: Thiazide Diuretic/ACE Inhibitor
Carafate	sucralfate	Ulcer

Brand Name	Generic Name(s)	Category
Cardene	nicardipine	Blood Pressure/Heart: Calcium Channel Blocker
Cardizem	diltiazem	Blood Pressure/Heart: Calcium Channel Blocker
Cardura	doxazosin	Blood Pressure: Peripheral Vasodilator
Cartrol	caretolol	Blood Pressure/Heart: Beta-Blocker
Catapres	clonidine	Blood Pressure: AntiAdrenergic
Ceclor	cefaclor	Antibiotic: Cephalosporin
Cedilandid-1	deslanoside	Cardiac Glycoside
Ceftin	cefuroxime	Antibiotic: Cephalosporin
Cefobid	cefoperazone	Antibiotic: Cephalosporin
Cefotan	cefotetan	Antibiotic: Cephalosporin
Cefzil	cefprozil	Antibiotic: Cephalosporin
Celestone	betamethasone	Adrenal Steroids: Glucocorticoid
Celontin	methsuximide	Anticonvulsant
Chardonna-2	belladonna alkaloids, phenobarbital	Ulcer/GI: Anticholinergic/ Barbiturate
Chlor-Trimeton	chlorpheniramine	Antihistamine
Chloromycetin	chloramphenicol	Antibiotic: Chloramphenicol
Choledyl	oxtriphylline	Asthma: Xanthine Bronchodilator
Choloxin	dextrothyroxine	Cholesteroil/Lipid Lowering
Chooz	calcium carbonate	Antacid
Cinobac	cinoxacin	Urinary Anti-Infective
Cipro	ciprofloxacin	Antibiotic: Fluoroquinolone
Citrucel	methylcellulose	Laxative: Bulk Fiber
Claritin	loratadine	Antihistamine: Nonsedating
Cleocin	clindamycin	Antibiotic: Lincosamide
Clinoril	sulindac	Analgesic: NSAID
Clozaril	clozapine	Antipsychotic
Cogentin	benztropine	Parkinsons: Anticholinergic
Cognex	tacrine	Dementia
Colace	docusate (dioctyl sodium sulfosuccinate, DSS)	Stool Softener

Brand Name	Generic Name(s)	Category
ColBenemid	probenecid, colchicine	Gout
Colestid	colestipol	Cholesteroil/Lipid Lowering
Coly-Mycin S	colistin	Antibiotic: Aminoglycoside
Combipres	chlorthalidone, clonidine	Blood Pressure: Thiazide Diuretic/AntiAdrenergic
Compazine	prochlorperazine	Antipsychotic: Phenothiazine
Cordarone	amiodarone	Arrhythmia
Corgard	nadolol	Blood Pressure/Heart: Beta-Blocker
Cortef	hydrocortisone	Adrenal Steroids: Glucocorticoids
Cortisol	hydrocortisone	Adrinal Steroids: Glucocorticoids
Cortone	cortisone	Adrenal Steroids: Glucocorticoids
Corzide	bendroflumethiazide, nadolol	Blood Pressure: Thiazide Diuretic/Beta-Blocker
Cotazym-S	digestive enzymes	Digestive Enzymes
Cotrim	sulfamethoxazole	Antibiotic: Sulfa/Trimethoprim
Coumadin	warfarin	Anticoagulant (“blood thinner”)
Cozaar	Iosartan	Blood Pressure: Angiotensin II Antagonist
Crixivan	indinavir	AntiViral
Crystodigin	digitoxin	Heart: Cardiac Glycoside
Cuprimine	penicillamine	Anti-Inflammatory
Cyanocobalamin	Vitamin B_{12}	Vitamin
Cyclan	cyclandelate	Blood Pressure/Heart: Peripheral Vasodilator
Cylert	pemoline	Stimulant
Cytomel	liothyronine	Thyroid Hormone
Cytotec	misoprostol	Ulcer
Cytovene	ganciclovir	Antiviral
Cytoxan	cyclophosphamide	Cancer: Nitrogen Mustard
Dalmane	flurazepam	Sedative: Benzodiazepine
Dantrium	dantrolene	Muscle Relaxant
Dapsone	dapsone	Leprosy
Daraprim	pyrimethamine	Malaria
Daricon	oxyphencyclimine	Ulcer/GI: Anticholinergic

Brand Name	Generic Name(s)	Category
Darvocet N	propoxyphene acetaminophen	Analgesic: Narcotic/ Acetaminophen
Darvon	propoxyphene	Analgesic: Narcotic
Darvon Compound	propoxyphene, aspirin, caffeine	Analgesic: Narcotic/Aspirin/ Caffeine
Daypro	oxaprozin	Nonnarcotic Analgesic: NSAID
Decadron	dexamethasone	Adrenal Steroids: Glucocorticoids
Declomycin	demeclocycline	Antibiotic: Tetracycline
Delta-Cortef	prednisolone	Adrenal Steroids: Glucocorticoids
Deltasone	prednisone	Adrenal Steroids: Glucocorticoids
Demadix	torsemide	Diuretic: Loop
Demerol	meperidine	Analgesic: Narcotic
Demulen	ethinyl estradiol, ethynodiol diacetate	Contraceptive (oral)
Depakene	valproic acid	Anticonvulsant
Depakote	valproic acid	Anticonvulsant
Deprol	meprobamate	Psychotherapeutic: AntiAnxiety/ AntiDepressant
Desoxyn	methamphetamine	Amphetamine
Desyrel	trazodone	Antidepressant
Dexacort	dexamethasone	Adrenal Steroids: Glucocorticoids
Dexedrine	dextroamphetamine	Amphetamine
DHE	dihydroergotamine	Migraine
DiaBeta	glyburide (glibenclamide)	Diabetes (oral): Sulfonylurea
Diabinese	chlorpropamide	Diabetes (oral): Sulfonylurea
Dicumarol	dicumarol	Anticoagulant (“blood thinner”)
Didrex	benzphetamine	Anorexiant: Amphetamine-like
Diflucan	fluconazole	Antifungal
Digitalis	cardiac glycosides:	Digoxin, Digitoxin, Deslanoside)
Dilantin	phenytoin	Anticonvulsant: Hydantoin
Dilaudid	hydromorphone	Analgesic: Narcotic
Dilor	dyphylline	Asthma: Xanthine Bronchodilator
Dilor G	dyphylline, guaifenesin	Asthma: Xanthine Bronchodilator/expectorant
Dimetane	brompheniramine	Antihistamine

Brand Name	Generic Name(s)	Category
Disalcid	salsalate	Analgesic: NSAID - Salicylate
Diucardin	hydroflumethiazide	Diuretic: Thiazide
Diupres	chlorothiazide reserpine	Blood Pressure: Thiazide Diuretic/Rauwolfia Derivative
Diuril	chlorothizide	Diuretic: Thiazide
Doan's (original)	magnesium salicylate	Analgesic: NSAID - Salicylate
Dolobid	diflunisal	Analgesic: NSAID - Salicylate
Dolophine	methadone	Analgesic: Narcotic
Donnagel	attapulgite	Antidiarrheal
Donnatal	atropine, scopolamine, hyoscyamine, phenobarbital	Ulcer/GI: Anticholinertgic/ Barbiturate
Dopar	levodopa	Parkinsons
Doral	quazepam	Sedative: Benzodiazepine
Doryx	doxycycline	Antibiotic: Tetracycline
Dr. Caldwell Laxative	senna	Laxative: Stimulant
Dulcolax	bisacodyl	Laxative: Stimulant
Durabolin	nandrolone	Anabolic Steroid
Duricef	cefadroxil	Antibiotic: Cephalosporin
Dyazide	hydrochlorothiazide, triamterene	Blood Pressure: Thiazide and Potassium-sparing Diuretics
Dycill	dicloxacillin	Antibiotic: Penicillin
Dymelor	acetohexamide	Diabetes (oral): Sulfonylurea
Dynabac	dirithromycin	Antibiotic: Macrolide
DynaCirc	isradipine	Blood Pressure/Heart: Calcium Channel Blocker
Dynapen	dicloxacillin	Antibiotic: Penicillin
Dyrenium	triamterene	Diuretic: Potassium-sparing
E-Mycin	erythromycin	Antibiotic: Macrolide
Edecrin	ethacrynic acid	Diuretic: Loop
EES	erythromycin	Antibiotic: Macrolide
Effexor	venlafaxine	Antidepressant
Efidac/24	pseudoephedrine	Decongestant
Elavil	amitryptyline	Antidepressant: Tricyclic

Brand Name	Generic Name(s)	Category
Eldepryl	selegiline	Parkinsons
Elixophyllin	theophylline	Asthma: Xanthine Brochodilator
Elixophyllin GG	theophylline, guaifenesin	Asthma: Xanthine Bronchodilator/Expectorant
Empirin/Codeine	codeine, aspirin	Analgesic: Narcotic/Aspirin
Endep	amitryptyline	Antidepressant: Tricyclic
Enduron	methyclothiazide	Diuretic: Thiazide
Enduronyl	methyclothiazide, deserpidine	Blood Pressure: Thiazide Diuretic
Enkaid	encainide	Arrhythmia
Enovid	norethynodrel, mestranol	Contraceptive (oral): Estrogen/ Progestin
Epsom Salt	magnesium sulfate	Laxative: Saline
Equanil	meprobamate	Antianxiety
Ergostat	ergotamine	Migraine
Ery-Tab	erythromycin	Antibiotic: Macrolide
Eryc	erythromycin	Antibiotic: Macrolide
EryPed	erythromycin	Antibiotic: Macrolide
Esgic	acetaminophen, caffeine, butalbital	Analgesic: Acetaminophen/ Caffeine/Barbiturate
Esidrix	hydrochlorothiazide	Diuretic: thiazide
Esimil	hydrochlorothiazide, guanethidine	Blood Pressure: Thiazide Diuretic/Peripheral Vasodilator
Eskalith	lithium	Antipsychotic
Estinyl	ethinyl estradiol	Estrogen
Estrace	estradiol	Estrogen
Estratab	estrogens (esterified)	Estrogen
Estrovis	quinestrol	Estrogen
Ethmozine	moricizine	Arrhythmic
Etrafon	perphenazine amitriptyline	Psychotherapeutic: Phenothiazine/ Tricyclic Antidepressant
Ex-Lax	phenolphthalein	Laxative: Stimulant
Exna	benzthiazide	Diuretic: Thiazide
Fansidar	sulfadoxine pyrimethamine	Malaria
Fastin	phentermine	Anorexiant: Amphetamine-like

Brand Name	Generic Name(s)	Category
Febatol	felbamate	Anticonvulsant
Feen-a-Mint	phenolphthalein	Laxative: Stimulant
Feldene	piroxicam	Analgesic: NSAID
Fioricet	acetaminophen caffeine, butalbital	Analgesic: Acetaminophen/ Caffeine/Barbiturate
Fioricet/Codeine	acetaminophen caffeine, butalbital, codeine	Analgesic: Acetaminophen/ Caffeine/Barbiturate/Narcotic
Fiorinal	aspirin, caffeine, butalbital	Analgesic: NSAID (salicylate)/ Caffeine/Barbiturate
Fiorinal/Codeine	aspirin, caffeine, butalbital, codeine	Analgesic: NSAID (salicylate)/ Caffeine/Barbiturate/Narcotic
Flagyl	metronidazole	Antifungal
Fletcher's Castoira	senna	Laxative: Stimulant
Flexeril	cyclobenzaprine	Muscle Relaxant
Floxin	ofloxacin	Antibiotic: Fluoroquinolone
Formula Q	quinine	Malaria
Frisium	clobazam	Antianxiety: Benzodiazepine
Fulvicin	griseofulvin	Antifungal
Furadantin	nitrofurantoin	Urinary Anti-Infective
Furoxone	furazolidone	Antibiotic
Gantanol	sulfamethoxazole	Antibiotic: Sulfa
Gantrisin	sulfisoxazole	Antibiotic: Sulfa
Gas-X	simethicone	Antiflatulent
Garamycin	gentamicin	Antibiotic: Aminoglycoside
Gaviscon	sodium bicarbonate alginic acid magnesium trisilicate	Antacid
Geocillin	carbenicillin	Antibiotic: Penicillin
Glucophage	metformin	Diabetes (oral): Biguanide
Glucotrol	glipizide	Diabetes (oral): Sulfonylurea
Grifulvin V	griseofulvin	Antifungal
Gris-PEG	griseofulvin	Antifungal
Grisactin	griseofulvin	Antifungal
Habritrol	nicotine	Smoking Deterrent

Brand Name	Generic Name(s)	Category
Halcion	triazolam	Sedative: Benzodiazepine
Haldol	haloperidol	Antipsychotic
Halotestin	fluoxymesterone	Androgen
Heparin	heparin	Anticoagulant ("blood thinner")
Hiprex	methenamine	Urinary Anti-Infective
Hismanal	astemizole	Antihistamine: Nonsedating
Hivid	zalcitabine (dideoxycytidine, DDC)	Antiviral
Humatin	paromomycin	Antibiotic: Aminoglycoside
Humulin	insulin	Diabetes (injection)
Hydergine	ergot alkaloids	Psychotherapeutic
Hydrocortone	hydrocortisone	Adrenal Steroid: Glucocorticoids
HydroDiuril	hydrochlorothiazide	Diuretic: Thiazide
Hydromox	quinethazone	Diuretic: Thiazide
Hydropres	hydrochlorothiazide reserpine	Blood Pressure: Thiazide Diuretic/Rauwolfia Derivative
Hygroton	chlorthalidone	Diuretic: Tiazide
Hylorel	guanadrel	Blood Pressure: Peripheral Vasodilator
Hytrin	terazosin	Blood Pressure: Peripheral Vasodilator
Hyzaar	hydrochlorothiazide losartan	Blood Pressure: Thiazide Diuretic/Angiotensen Antagonist
Iletin	insulin	Diabetes (injection)
Ilosone	erythromycin	Antibiotic: Macrolide
Imdur	isosorbide mononitrate	Angina: Nitrate
Imitrex	sumatriptan	Migraine
Imodium	loperamide	Antidiarrheal
Inderal	propranolol	Blood Pressure/Heart: Beta-blocker
Inderide	hydrochlorothiazide propranolol	Blood Pressure: Thiazide Diuretic/Beta-blocker
Indocin	indomethacin	Analgesic: NSAID
Insulin	insulin	Diabetes (injection)
Inversine	mecamylamine	Blood Pressure: Ganglionic Blocker

Brand Name	Generic Name(s)	Category
Invirase	saquinavir	AntiViral
Ionamin	phentermine	Anorexiant: Amphetamine-like
Ismelin	quanethidine	Blood Pressure: Peripheral Vasodilator
Isocarboxazid	isocarboxazid	Antidepressant: MAOI
Isoptin	verapamil	Blood Pressure/Heart: Calcium Channel Blocker
Isordil	isorbide dinitrate	Angina: Nitrate
Isuprel	isoproterenol	Asthma: Bronchodilator - Sympathomimetic
Kantrex	kanamycin	Antibiotic: Aminoglycoside
Kaopectate	kaolin pectin	Antidiarrheal
Kayexalate	sodium polystyrene sulfonate	Potassium Removal
Keflex	cephalexin	Antibiotic: Cephalosporin
Keftab	cephalexin	Antibiotic: Cephalosporin
Kefurox	cefuroxime	Antibiotic: Cephalosporin
Kemadrin	procyclidine	Parkinsons: Anticholinergic
Kenacort	triamcinolone	Adrenal Steroids: Glucocorticoids
Kerlone	betaxolol	Blood Pressure/Heart: Beta-Blocker
Klonopin	clonazepam	Anticonvulsant: Benzodiazepine
Kondremul	mineral oil	Laxative: Emolient
Ku-Zyme	digestive enzymes	Digestive Enzymes
Lamictal	lamotrigine	Anticonvulsant
Laniazid	isoniazid	Tuberculosis
Lanoxicap	digoxin	Heart: Cardiac Glycoside
Lanoxin	digoxin	Heart: Cardiac Glycoside
Larium	mefloquine	Malaria
Lasix	furosemide	Diuretic: Loop
Ledercillin VK	penicillin V	Antibiotic: Pencillin
Lescol	fluvastatin	Cholesteroil/Lipid Lowering
Levatol	penbutolol	Blood Pressure/Heart: Beta-blocker
Levsin	hyoscycamine	Ulcer/GI: Antichoninergic

Brand Name	Generic Name(s)	Category
Levsin PB	hyoscyamine phenobarbital	Ulcer/GI: Antichoninergic/ Barbiturate
Librax	chlordiazepoxide clidinium	Ulcer/GI: Benzodiazepine/ Anticholinergic
Libritab	chlordiazepoxide	Antianxiety: Benzodiazepine
Librium	chlordiazepoxide	Antianxiety: Benzodiazepine
Limbitrol	chlordiazepoxide amitriptyline	Psychotherapeutic: Benzodiazepine/ Tricyclic Antidepressant
Lincocin	lincomycin	Antibiotic: Lincosamide
Lioresal	baclofen	Muscle Relaxant
Lo/Ovral	ethinyl estradiol, noregestrel	Contraceptive (oral): Estrogen/ Progestin
Lodine	etodolac	Analgesic: NSAID
Lodosyn	carbidopa	Parkinsons
Loestrin	ethinyl estradiol, norethindrone	Contraceptive (oral): Estrogen/ Progestin
Lomotil	diphenoxylate atropine	Antidiarrheal: Narcotic/ Antichonlinergic
Loniten	minoxidil	Blood Pressure: Vasodilator
Lopid	gemfibrazil	Cholesterol/Lipid Lowering
Lopressor	metoprolol	Blood Pressure/Heart: Beta-blocker
Lopressor HCT	metoprolol	Blood Pressure/Heart: Beta-blocker/Thiazide Diuretic
Lorabid	loracarbef	Antibiotic: Cephalosporin
Lorelco	probucol	Cholesterol/Lipid Lowering
Lortab	hydrocodone acetaminophen	Analgesic: Narcotic/ acetaminophen
Lotensin	benazepril	Blood Pressure: ACE Inhibitor
Lotensin HCT	benazepril hydrochlorothiazide	Blood Pressure: ACE Inhibitor/ Thiazide Diuretic
Lotrel	benazepril amlodipine	Blood Pressure: ACE Inhibitor/ Calcium Channel Blocker
Levo-Dromoran	levorphanol	Analgesic: Narcotic
Loxapine	loxitane	Antipsychotic
Lozol	indapamide	Diuretic: Thiazide

Brand Name	Generic Name(s)	Category
Ludiomil	maprotiline	Antidepressant: Tetracyclic
Lufyllin	dyphylline	Asthma: Xanthine Bronchodilator
Lufyllin GG	dyphylline guaifenesin	Asthma: Xanthine Bronchodilator/Expectorant
Luminal	phenobarbital	Sedative: Barbiturate
Luvox	fluvoxamine	Antidepressant: SSRI
Maalox	aluminum hydroxide magnesium hydroxide	Antacid
Mag Citrate	magnesium citrate	Laxative: Saline
Mag-Ox	magnesium oxide	Antacid
Mandelamine	methenamine	Urinary Anti-infective
Mandol	cefamandole	Antibiotic: Cephalosporin
Marax	theophylline ephedrine	Asthma: Xanthine Bronchodilator/Decongestant
Marezine	cyclizine	Motion Sickness: Antihistamine
Marinol	dronabinol	Marijuana-like agent
Matulane	procarbazine	Cancer
Maxair	pirbuterol	Asthma: Sympathomimetic Bronchodilator
Maxaquin	lomefloxacin	Antibiotic: Fluoroquinolone
Maxzide	hydrochlorothiazide triamterene	Diuretic: Thiazide/Potassium-sparing
Mazanor	mazindol	Anorexient: Amphetamine-like
Mebaral	mephobarbital	Sedative: Barbiturate
Meclomen	meclofenamate	Analgesic: NSAID
Medrol	methylprednisolone	Adrenal Steroid: Glucocorticoid
Mellaril	thioridazine	Antipsychotic: Phenothiazine
Menest	estrogens	Estrogen
Mepergan Fortis	meperidine promethazine	Analgesic: Narcotic/ Phenothiazine
Mepron	atovaquone	Antiprotozoal
Mesantoin	mephenytoin	Anticonvulsant: Hydantoin
Metahydrin	trichlormethiazide	Diuretic: Thiazide
Metamucil	psyllium	Laxative: Bulk
Metaprel	metaproterenol	Asthma: Sympathomimetic Bronchodilator

Brand Name	Generic Name(s)	Category
Meticorten	prednisone	Adrenal Steroid: Glucocorticoid
Mevacor	lovastatin	Cholesterol/Lipid Lowering
Mexitil	mexiletine	Arrhythmia
Micronase	glyburide (glibenclamide)	Diabetes: Sulfonylurea
Midamor	amiloride	Diuretic: Potassium-sparing
Midol IB	ibuprofen	Anlgesic: NSAID
Midrin	acetaminophen isometheptene dichloralphenazone	Mirgrain
Milk of Magnesia	magnesium hydroxide	Antacid (lower doses); Laxative (higher doses)
Milkinol	mineral oil	Laxative: Emolient
Milontin	phensuximde	Anticonvulsant
Miltown	meprobamate	Antianxiety
Minipres	prazosin	Blood Pressure: Peripheral Vasodilator
Minizide	prazosin polythiazide	Blood Pressure: Peripheral Vasodilator/Thiazide Diuretic
Minocin	minocycline	Antibiotic: Tetracycline
Moban	molindone	Antipsychotic
Mobidin	magnesium salicylate	Analgesic: NSAID (salicylate)
Modane	phenolphthalein	Laxative: Stimulant
Moderil	rescinnamine	Blood Pressure: Rauwolfia Derivative
Modicon	ethinyl estradiol, norethindrome	Contraceptive (oral): Estrogen/Progestin
Moduretic	hydrochlorothiazide amiloride	Diuretic: Thiazide and Potassium-sparing
Monopril	fosinopril	Blood Pressure: ACE Inhibitor
Motrin	ibuprofen	Analgesic: NSAID
Moxalactam	moxalactam	Antibiotic: Cephalosporin
MS Contin	morphine	Analgesic: Narcotic
Myambutol	ethambutol	Tuberculosis
Mycifradin	neomycin	Antibiotic: Aminoglycoside
Mycobutin	rifabutin	Tuberculosis

Brand Name	Generic Name(s)	Category
Mycostatin	nystatin	Antifungal
Mylanta	aluminum hydroxide magnesium hydroxide	Antacid
Mylanta Gas	simethicone	Antiflatulent
Mylicon	simethicone	Antiflatulent
Mysoline	primidone	Anticonvulsant
Nalfon	fenoprofen	Analgesic: NSAID
Naprosyn	naproxen	Analgesic: NSAID
Naqua	trichlormethiazide	Diuretic: Thiazide
Nardil	phenelzine	Antidepressant: MAOI
Naturetin	bendroflumethiazide	Diuretic: Thiazide
Navane	thiothizene	Antipsychotic
Nebcin	tobramycin	Antibiotic: Aminoglycoside
NegGram	nalidixic acid	Urinary Anti-infective
Nembutal	pentobarbital	Sedative: Barbiturate
Neo-Synephrine	phenylephrine	Decongestant
Neoral	cyclosporine	Immunosuppressive
Neurontin	gabapentin	Anticonvulsant
Niacin	Vitamin B_3	Vitamin
Nicoderm	nicotine	Smoking Deterrent
Nicorette	nicotine	Smoking Deterrent
Nicotrol	nicotine	Smoking Deterrent
Nilstat	nystatin	Antifungal
Nimotop	nimodipine	Blood Pressure/Heart: Calcium Channel Blocker
Nitro-Bid	nitroglycerin	Angina: Nitrate
Nitro-Dur	nitroglycerin	Angina: Nitrate
Nitrogard	nitroglycerin	Angina: Nitrate
Nitroglyn	nitroglycerin	Angina: Nitrate
Nitrostat	nitroglycerin	Angina: Nitrate
Nizoral	ketoconazole	Antifungal
Nolahist	phenindamine	Antihistamine
Nordette	ethinyl estradiol, levonorgestrel	Contraceptive (oral): Estrogen/Progestin
Norflex	orphenadrine	Muscle Relaxant

Brand Name	Generic Name(s)	Category
Norgesic	orphenadrine aspirin, caffeine	Muscle Relaxant/Analgesic
Norinyl	ethinyl estradiol, norethindrone	Contraceptive (oral): Estrogen/Progestin
Norlutin	norethindrone	Progestin
Normodyne	labetalol	Alpha/Beta-Blocker
Noroxin	norflxacin	Antibiotic: Fluoroquinolone
Norpace	disopyramide	Arrhythmia
Norpramin	desipramine	Antidepressant: Tricyclic
Norvasc	amlodipine	Blood Pressure/Heart: Calcium Channel Blocker
Novafed	pseudoephedrine	Decongestant
Novolin	insulin	Diabetes (injection)
Numorphan	oxymorphone	Analgesic: Narcotic
Nuprin	ibuprofen	Analgesic: NSAID
Nydrazid	isoniazid	Tuberculosis
Ogen	estropipate	Estrogen
Omnipen	ampicillin	Antibiotic: Penicillin
Oncovin	vincristine	Cancer: Mitotic Inhibitor
Optimine	azatadine	Antihistamine
Orap	pimozide	Antipsychotic
Oretic	hydrochlorothiazide	Diuretic: Thiazide
Oreton Methyl	methyltestosterone	Androgen
Orinase	tolbutamide	Diabetes: Sulfonylruea
Ortho-Novum	norethindrone, mestranol	Contraceptive (oral): Estrogen/Progestin
Orudis	ketoprofen	Analgesic: NSAID
Oruvail	ketoprofen	Analgesic: NSAID
Otrivin	xylometazoline	Decongestant
Ovcon	ethinyl estradiol, norethindrone	Contraceptive (oral): Estrogen/Progestin
Ovral	ethinyl estradiol, norgestrel	Contraceptive (oral): Estrogen/Progestin
Oxandrin	oxandrolone	Anaholic Steroid
Oxyphenbutazone	oxyphenbutazone	Analgesic: NSAID

Brand Name	Generic Name(s)	Category
PABA	Para-Aminobenzoid Acid	Vitamin
Pamelor	nortriptyline	Antidepressant: Tricyclic
Pamine	methscopolamine	Ulcer/GI: Anticholinergic
Panmycin	tetracycline	Antibiotic: Tetracycline
Parafon Forte DSC	chlorzoxazone	Muscle Relaxant
Paral	paraldehyde	Sedative
Para-Aminosalicylic Acid (PAS)	para-aminosalicylic acid	Tuberculosis
Parlodel	bromocriptine	Parkinsons
Parnate	tranylcypromine	Antidepressant: MAOI
Parsidol	ethopropazine	Parkinsons: Anticholinergic
Pathilon	tridihexethyl	Ulcer/GI: Anticholinergic
Pathocil	dicloxacillin	Antibiotic: Penicillin
Pavabid	papaverine	Peripheral Vasodilator
Paxil	paroxetine	Antidepressant: SSRI
PBZ	tripelennamine	Antihistamine
PCE	erythromycin	Antibiotic: Macrolide
Pediazole	erythromycin	Antibiotic: Macrolide/Sulfa
Peganone	ethotoin	Anticonvulsant: Hydantoin
Pen Vee K	penicillin V	Antibiotic: PCN
Pen-V	penicillin V	Antibiotic: PCN
Penetrex	enoxacin	Antibiotic: Fluoroquinolones
Pentam	pentamidine	Antiprotozoal
Pentids	penicillin G	Antibiotic: Penicillin
Pepcid	famotidine	H2 Blockers
Pepto-Bismol	bismuth subsalicylate	Antidiarrheal/Salicylate
Percocet	oxycodone acetaminophen	Analgesic: Narcotic/ Acetaminophen
Percodan	oxycodone aspirin	Analgesic: Narcotic/Aspirin
Perdiem	psyllium	Laxative: Bulk
Periactin	cyproheptadinc	Antihistamine
Peridex	chlorhexidine	Antiseptic Oral Rinse

Brand Name	Generic Name(s)	Category
PerioGard	chlorhexidine	Antiseptic Oral Rinse
Permax	pergolide	Parkinsons
Permitil	fluphenazine	Antipsychotic: phenothiazine
Phazyme	simethicone	Antiflatulent
Phenaphen/ Codeine	codeine acetaminophen	Analgesic: Narcotic/ Acetaminophen
Phenergan	promethazine	Antihistamine/Phenothiazine
Phenurone	phenacemide	Anticonvulsant
PhosLo	calcium acetate	Nutritional Supplement: Mineral
Phrenilin	acetaminophen caffeine	Analgesic: Acetaminophen/ Caffeine/Barbiturate
Placidyl	ethchlorvynol	Sedative
Plaquenil	hydroxychloroquine	Malaria/Antirheumatic
Platinol	cisplatin	Cancer: Alkylating Agent
Plendil	felodipine	Blood Pressure/Heart: Calcium Channel Blocker
Polaramine	dexchlorpheniramine	Antihistamine
Poly-Histine	pheniramine pyrilamine phenyltoloxamine	Antihistamine Combination
Polycillin	ampicillin	Antibiotic: Penicillin
Polymox	amoxicillin	Antibiotic: Penicillin
Pondimin	fenfluramine	Anorexiant: Amphetamine-like
Ponstel	mefanamic acid	Analgesic: NSAID
Pravachol	pravastatin	Cholesterol/Lip Lowering
Prelu-2	phendimetrazine	Anorexiant: Amphetamine-like
Premarin	estrogen(conjugated)	Estrogen
Prevacid	lansoprazole	Ulcer/GI
Prilosec	omeprazole	Ulcer/GI
Primatene	theophylline ephedrine	Asthma: Xanthine Bronchodilator/ Decongestant
Primatene Mist	ephedrin	Asthma: Decongestant
Principen	ampicillin	Antibiotic: Penicillin
Prinivil	lisinopril	Blood Pressure: ACE Inhibitor
Prinzide	lisinopril hydrochlorothiazide	Blood Pressure: ACE Inhibitor/ Thiazide Diuretic

Brand Name	Generic Name(s)	Category
Privine	naphazoline	Decongestant
Pro-Banthine	propantheline	Ulcer/GI: Anticholinergic
Procan SR	procainamide	Arrhythmic
Procardia	nifedipine	Blood Pressure/Heart: Calcium Channel Blocker
Prolixin	fluphenazine	Antipsychotic: Phenothiazine
Proloprim	trimethoprim	Antibiotic
Pronestyl	procainamide	Arrhythmic
Propylthiouracil	propylthiouracil	Antithyroid
ProSom	estazolam	Sedative: Benzodiazepine
ProStep	nicotine	Smoking Deterrent
Prostaphlin	oxacillin	Antibiotic: Penicillin
Proventil	albuterol	Sympathomimetic Bronchodilator
Provera	medroxyprogesterone	Progestin
Prozac	fluoxetine	Antidepressant: SSRI
Pyridoxine	vitamin B_6	Vitamin
Quarzan	clidiuium	Ulcer/GI: Anticholinergic
Questran	cholestyramine	Cholesterol/Lipid Lowering
Quibron	theophylline guaifenesin	Asthma: Xanthine Bronchodilator/ Expectorant
Quibron-T	theophylline	Xanthine Bronchodilator
Quinacrine	quinacrine	Antimalarial
Quinamm	quinine	Antimalarial
Quinora	quinidine	Arrhythmia
Raudixin	rauwolfia	Blood Pressure: Peripheral Vasodilator
Rauzide	rauwolfia bendroflumethiazide	Blood Pressure: Peripheral Vasodilator/Thiazide Diuretic
Reglan	metoclopramide	Nausea
Regroton	reserpine chlorthalidone	Blood Pressure: Peripheral Vasodilator/Thiazide Diuretic
Relafen	nabumetone	Analgesic: NSAID
Renese	polythiazide	Diuretic: Thiazide
Renese R	polythiazide reserpinc	Blood Pressure: Thiazide Diuretic/Peripheral Vasodilator

Brand Name	Generic Name(s)	Category
Renoquid	sulfacytine	Antibiotic: Sulfa
Respbid	theophylline	Asthma: Xanthine Bronchodilator
Restoril	temazepam	Sedative: Benzodiazepine
Retinol	vitamin A	Vitamin
Retrovir	zidovudine (azidothymidine, AZT; Compound S)	AntiViral
Rheumatrex	methotrexate	Antirheumatic
Riboflavin	Vitamin B_2	Vitamin
Rifadin	rifampin	Tuberculosis
Rifamate	isoniazid rifampin	Tuberculosis
Rifater	isoniazid rifampin pyrazinamide	Tuberculosis
Rimactane	rifampin	Tuberculosis
Rimactane/INH	isoniazid rifampin	Tuberculosis
Riopan	magaldrate	Antacid
Risperdal	risperidone	Antipsychotic
Ritalin	methylphenidate	Stimulant
Robaxin	methocarbamol	Muscle Relaxant
Robaxisal	methocarbamol aspirin	Muscle Relaxant/NSAID (salicylate)
Robicillin VK	penicillin V	Antibiotic: Penicillin
Robinul	glycopyrrolate	Ulcer/GI: Anticholinergic
Rubex	doxorubicin	Antibiotic: Anthracyclkine
Rythmol	propafenone	Arrhythmia
Salutensin	hydroflumethiazide reserpine	Blood Pressure: Thiazide Diuretic/Rauwolfia Derivative
Sandimmune	cyclosporine	Immunosuppressive
Sanorex	mazindol	Anorexiant: Amphetamine-like
Sansert	methysergide	Migraine
Seconal	secobarbital	Sedative: Barbiturate
Sectral	acebutolol	Blood Pressure/Heart: Beta-Blocker

Brand Name	Generic Name(s)	Category
Seldane	terfenadine	Antihistamine: nonsedating
Senokot	senna	Laxative: Stimulant
Septra	sulfamethoxazole trimethoprim	Antibiotic: Sulfa/Trimethoprim
Ser-Ap-Es	hydrochlorothiazide reserpine hydralazine	Blood Pressure: Thiazide Diuretic/ Rauwolfia Derivative/Vasodilator
Serax	oxazepam	Antianxiety: Benzodiazepine
Serentil	mesoridazine	Antipsychotic: Phenothiazine
Seromycin	cycloserine	Tuberculosis
Serutan	psyllium	Laxative: Bulk
Serzone	nefazodone	Antidepressant
Sinemet	levodopa carbidopa	Parkinsons
Sinequan	doxepin	Antidepressant: Tricyclic
Skelaxin	metaxalone	Muscle Relaxant
Slo-Phyllin	theophylline	Asthma: Xanthine Bronchodilator
Slo-Phyllin GG	theophylline guaifenesin	Asthma: Xanthine Bronchodilator/Expectorant
Soma	carisoprodol	Muscle Relaxant
Soma Compound	carisoprodol aspirin	Muscle Relaxant/NSAID (salicylate)
Sorbitrate	isosorbide dinitrate	Angina: Nitrate
Sparine	promazine	Antipsychotic: Phenothiazine
Spectrobid	bacampicillin	Antibiotic: Penicillin
Sporanox	itraconazole	Antifungal
Stadol	butorphanol	Analgesic: Narcotic
Stelazine	trifluoperazine	Antipsychotic: Phenothiazine
Streptomycin	streptomycin	Antibiotic: Aminoglycoside
Sudafed	pseudoephedrine	Decongestant (sympathomimetic)
Sumycin	tetracycline	Antibiotic: Tetracycline
Suprax	cefixime	Antibiotic: Cephalosporin
Surmontil	trimipramine	Antidepressant: Tricyclic
Sustaire	theophylline	Asthma: Xanthine Bronchodilator
Symmetrel	amantadine	Parkinsons

Brand Name	Generic Name(s)	Category
Synalgos DC	codeine, aspirin	Analgesic: Narcotic/NSAID (salicylate)/caffeine
Synthroid	levothyroxine (thyroxine)	Thyroid Hormone
Tacaryl	methdilazine	Antihistamine/Phenothiazine
Tace	chlorotrianisene	Estrogen
Tagamet	cimetidine	H2 Blocker
Talacen	pentazocine acetaminophen	Analgesic: Narcotic/Acetaminophen
Talwin	pentazocine	Analgesic: Narcotic
Talwin Compound	pentazocine aspirin	Analgesic: Narcotic/NSAID (salicylate)
Tambocor	flecainide	Arrhythmia
Tao	erythromycin	Antibiotic: Macrolide
Tavist	clemastine	Antihistamine
Tegopen	cloxacillin	Antibiotic: Penicillin
Tegretol	carbamazepine	Anticonvulsant
Teldrin	chlorpheniramine	Antihistamine
Tenex	guanfacine	Blood Pressure: Central Acting
Tenoretic	chlorthalidone atenolol	Blood Pressure: Thiazide Diuretic/Beta-Blocker
Tenormin	atenolol	Blood Pressure/Heart: Beta-Blocker
Tenuate	diethylpropion	Anorexiant: Amphetamine-like
Tepanil	diethylpropion	Anorexiant: Amphetamine-like
Terramycin	oxytetracycline	Antibiotic: Tetracycline
Tessalon Perles	benzonatate	Cough Suppressant: Anesthetic
Theo-24	theophylline	Asthma: Xanthine Bronchodilator
Theo-Dur	theophylline	Asthma: Xanthine Bronchodilator
Theobid	theophylline	Asthma: Xanthine Bronchodilator
Theolair	theophylline	Asthma: Xanthine Bronchodilator
Theovent	theophylline	Asthma: Xanthine Bronchodilator
Thiamine	vitamin B_1	Vitamin
Thiosulfil Forte	sulfamethizole	Antibiotic: Sulfa
Thorazine	chlorpromazine	Antipsychotic: Phenothiazine

Brand Name	Generic Name(s)	Category
Thyrar	thyroid	Thyroid Hormone
Thyrolar	liotrix	Thyroid Hormone
Ticlid	ticlopidine	Stroke Prevention
Tigan	trimethobenzamide	Nausea: Anticholinergic
Timolide	hydrochlorothiazide timolol	Blood Pressure: Thiazide Diuretic/Beta-blocker
Tindal	acetophenazine	Antipsychotic: Phenothiazine
Tofranil	imipramine	Antidepressant: Tricyclic
Tolectin	tolmetin	Analgesic: NSAID
Tolinase	tolazamide	Diabetes (oral): Sulfonylurea
Tonocard	tocainide	Arrhythmia
Toradol	ketorolac	Analgesic: NSAID
Totacillin	ampicillin	Antibiotic: Penicillin
Trancopal	chlormezanone	Antianxiety
Trandate	labetalol	Blood Pressure/Heart: Alpha/ Beta-blocker
Transderm-Nitro	nitroglycerin	Angina: Nitrate
Transderm-Scop	scopolamine	Motion Sickness: Anticholinergic
Tranxene	clorazepate	Antianxiety: Benzodiazepine
Trecator-SC	ethionamide	Tuberculosis
Trimpex	trimethoprim	Antibiotic
Tri-Norinyl	ethinyl estradiol norethindrone	Contraceptive (oral): Estrogen/ Progestin
Triavil	perphenazine, amitriptyline	Psychotherapeutic: Phenothiazine/Tricyclic
Tridione	trimethadione	Anticonvulsant
Trilafon	perphenazine	Antipsychotic: Phenothiazine
Trilisate	choline salicylate magnesium salicylate	Analgesic: NSAID (salicylate)
Tri-Phasil	ethinyl estradiol levonorgastrel	Contraceptive (oral): Estrogen/ Progestin
Tums	calcium carbonate	Antacid
Tylenol/Codeine	codeine acetaminophen	Analgesic: Narcotic/ Acetaminophen
Tylox	oxycodone acetaminophen	Analgesic: Narcotic/ Acetaminophen

Brand Name	Generic Name(s)	Category
Tyzine	tetrahydrozoline	Decongestant (sympathomimetic)
Ultracef	cefadroxil	Antibiotic: Cephalosporin
Ultram	tramadol	Analgesic: Miscellaneous
Unipen	nafcillin	Antibiotic: Penicillin
Univasc	moexipril	Blood Pressure: ACE Inhibitor
Urex	methenamine	Urinary Anti-infective
Urobiotic	oxytetracycline sulfamethizole	Antibiotic: Tetracycline/Sulfa
V-Cillin K	penicillin V	Antibiotic: Penicillin
Valium	diazepam	AntiAnxiety: Benzodiazepine
Vanceril	beclomethasone	Asthma/Adrenal Steroid: Corticosteroid
Vancocin	vancomycin	Antibiotic: Miscellaneous
Vantin	cefpodoxime	Antibiotic: Cephalosporin
Vascor	bepridil	Blood Pressure/Heart: Calcium Channel Blocker
Vaseretic	hydrochlorothiazide enalapril	Blood Pressure: Thiazide Diuretic/ACE Inhibitor
Vasodilan	isoxsuprine	Peripheral Vasodilator
Vasotec	enalapril	Blood Pressure: ACE Inhibitor
Veetids	penicillin V	Antibiotic: Penicillin
Velosef	cephradine	Antibiotic: Cephalosporin
Velosulin	insulin	Diabetes (injection)
Ventolin	albuterol	Asthma: Sympathomimetic Bronchodilator
Versed	midazolam	Anesthetic: Benzodiazepine
Vesprin	triflupromazine	Antipsychotic: Phenothiazine
Vibra-Tabs	doxycycline	Antibiotic: Tetracycline
Vibramycin	doxycycline	Antibiotic: Tetracycline
Vicodin	hydrocodone acetaminophen	Analgesic: Narcotic/ Acetaminophen
Videx	didanosine (DDI; dideoxyinosine)	Antiviral
Viokase	digestive enzymes	Digestive Enzymes
Visken	pindolol	Blood Pressure/Heart: Beta-blocker

Brand Name	Generic Name(s)	Category
Vistaril	hydroxyzine	Antiznxiety: Antihistamine
Vitamin A	retinol	Vitamin
Vitamin B_1	thiamine	Vitamin
Vitamin B_2	riboflavin	Vitamin
Vitamin B_3	niacin (nicotinic acid)	Vitamin
Vitamin B_5	calcium pantothenate (pantothenic acid)	Vitamin
Vitamin B_6	pyridoxine	Vitamin
Vitamin B_{12}	cyanocobalamin	Vitamin
Vitamin C	ascorbic acid	Vitamin
Vitamin D	ergocalciferol (cholecalciferol)	Vitamin
Vitamin D_2	ergocalciferol	Vitamin
Vitamin D_3	cholecalciferol	Vitamin
Vitamin E	tocopherol	Vitamin
Vitamin P	bioflavonoids	Vitamin
Vivactil	protriptyline	Antidepressant: Tricyclic
Voltaren	diclofenac	Analgesic: NSAID
Vontrol	diphenidol	Nausea: Anticholinergic
Wellbutin	bupropion	Antidepressant
Wigraine	ergotamine, caffeine	Migraine
Winstrol	stanozolol	Anabolic Steroid
Wygesic	propoxyphene acetaminophen	Analgesic: Narcotic/ Acetaminophen
Wymox	amoxicillin	Antibiotic: Penicillin
Wytensen	guanabenz	Blood Pressure: Central Acting
Xanax	alprazolam	Antianxiety: Benzodiazepine
Zantac	ranitidine	H2 Blockers
Zarontin	ethosuximide	Anticonvulsant
Zaroxolyn	metolazone	Diuretic: Thiazide
Zebeta	bisoprolol	Blood Pressure/Heart: Beta-blocker
Zerit	stavudine	Antiviral
Zestoretic	hydrochlorothiazide, lisinopril	Blood Pressure: Thiazide Diuretic/ACE Inhibitor

Brand Name	Generic Name(s)	Category
Zestril	lisinopril	Blood Pressure/Heart: ACE Inhibitor
Ziac	hydrochlorothiazide, bisoprolol	Blood Pressure: Thiazide Diuretic/Beta-blocker
Zinacef	cefuroxime	Antibiotic: Cephalosporin
Zithromax	azithromycin	Antibiotic: Macrolide
Zocor	simvastatin	Cholesterol/Lipid Lowering
Zofran	ondansetron	Nausea
Zoloft	sertraline	Antidepressant: SSRI
Zyloprim	allopurinal	Gout

References

Bauwens, Eleanor, and Clemmons, Cindy. "Foods that Foil Drugs." *RN,* (September 1978), pp 79-81.

Tuttle, C. Brian. "Harmony with Drugs and Food." *CMA Journal,* (May 15 1982), pp. 1161-1162.

Lamy, Peter P. "Effects of Diet and Nutrition on Drug Therapy." *Journal of the American Geriatrics Society,* (November 1982), pp. S99-S112.

"Food Can Help, Delay or Reduce Drug Absorption." *Pharmacy Times,* (October 1982), pp. 52 ff. citing Welling, P.G., "Influence of Food and Diet on Gastrointestinal Absorption." A Review, *Journal of Pharmacokinetics and Biopharmaceutics,* Vol. 5, (1977), pp. 291-334.

Hazards Of Medication (2nd ed.), Lippincott, Philadelphia, (1978), pp. 399-408.

Durgin, Jane M. "Drug/Food Interactions." *Pharmacy Times,* (May 1980), pp. 32-40.

Bennett, Jerry A. "Drug-Food Interactions: A Guide for the Community Pharmacist." *The Apothecary,* (May/June 1977), pp. 8 ff.

Christakis, George. "Part II: Drug Interactions—Nutrients, Vitamins, Foods." *Pharmacy Times,* (November 1983), pp. 68 ff.

"Food and Drug Interactions." *FDA Consumer,* U.S. Dept. of Health, Education and Welfare, Public Health Service, FDA, Office of Public Affairs, (March 1978).

Bergman, H. David. "Effect of food on the bioavailability of orally administered drugs." *Hospital Formulary,* (April 1980), pp. 295-301.

Stanaszek, Walter F. "Food-Drug Interactions." C.E. Materials, School of Pharmacy, University of Oklahoma Health Sciences Center.

Powell, Michael F. and Lamy, Peter P. "Drug-Dietary Incompatibilities: II. Effects on Drug Therapy." *Hospital Formulary,* (December 1977), pp. 870-874.

Smith, Christine Hamilton, and Bidlack, Wayne R. "Dietary concerns associated with the use of medications." *Journal of the American Dietetic Association,* Vol. 84, No. 8, (August 1984), pp. 901-914.

Keithley, Joyce K., and O'Donnell, James. "Look out for these drug-nutrient interactions." *Nursing,* (February 1986), pp. 42-43.

Christakis, George, and Christakis, Paul. "Drug Interactions—Nutrients, Vitamins, Food." *Pharmacy Times,* (March 1986), pp. 51-55.

D'Arcy, P.F and McElnay, James C. "Drug-Antacid Interactions: Assessment of Clinical Importance." *Drug Intelligence and Clinical Pharmacy,* (July/Aug 1987), pp. 607-617.

"Advances in the Diagnosis and Management of Depression." *American Pharmacy,* Vol. NS28, No. 2, (February 1988), pp. 33-37.

Terrell, Christine L. and Hermans, Paul E. "Antifungal Agents Used for Deep-Seated Mycotic Infections." *Mayo Clin Proc,* (December 1987), pp. 1116-1128.

Clary, Cathryn and Schweizer, Edward. "Treatment of MAOI Crisis with Sublingual Nifedipine." *Journal of Clinical Psychiatry,* (June 1987), pp. 249-250.

Milne, D.B., et. al. "Metabolism of Ethanol in Postmenopausal Women Fed a Diet Marginal in Zinc." USDA-ARS, Grand Forks Human Nutrition Research Center, Grand Forks, ND.

Greenstein, Gary. "Chlorhexidine Use." *Journal of the American Dental Association,* (March 1987), p. 292.

Garabediajn-Ruffalo, Susan M. and Ruffalo, Richard L. "Drug and Nutrient Interactions." *AFP,* (February 1986), pp. 165-174.

Solomons, Noel W. "Competitive Interaction of Iron and Zinc in the Diet: Consequences for Human Nutrition." American Institute of Nutrition, (1986), pp. 927-935.

"Diet and Headache." National Migraine Foundation, Chicago, Ill.

Jann, Michael W.; Bean, Johnnie; and Fidone, George S. "Interaction of Dietary Pudding with Phenytoin." *Pediatrics,* Vol. 78, No. 5, (November, 1986), pp. 952-953.

Roe, Daphne A. "Drug-Nutrient Interactions in the Elderly." *Geriatrics,* Vol. 41, No. 3, (March 1986), pp. 57 ff.

Valli, C., et. al. "Interaction of Nutrients with Antacids: A Complication during Enteral Feeding." *The Lancet,* (March 29, 1986), pp. 747-748.

Hathcock, John N. "Metabolic Mechanisms of Drug-Nutrient Interactions." Federation Proceedings, Vol. 44, No. 1, PT. 1, (January, 1985), pp. 124-129, from the Symposium *Metabolic Interactions of Nutrition and Drugs* presented by the American Institute of Nutrition at the 67th Annual Meeting of the Federation of American Societies for Experimental Biology, Chicago, Ill., (April 11, 1983).

Ovesen, L; Lyduch, S; and Idorn, M.L. "The Effect of Brussel Sprouts on Warfarin Pharmacokinetics." Abstract cited in *Clinical Pharmacology and Therapeutics,* (February 1987), p. 246.

Bernstein, Jerrold G. and Bernstein, David B. "Psychotropic-Related Weight Gain—What Causes It, What to Do About It." *Drug Therapy,* (April 1987), pp. 109-119.

Hayes, J.R. and Borzelleca, J.F. "Nutrient Interaction with Drugs and Other Xenobiotics." *Journal of The American Dietetic Association,* (March, 1985), pp. 335-339.

The Pharmacological Basis of Therapeutics 6th ed. Alfred G. Gilman, Louis S. Goodman, Editors. MacMillan Publishing Co., New York, (1980).

Abernathy, Rosalind S. "Applesauce and Isoniazid" [letter], *Pediatrics,* Vol. 79., No. 3, (March, 1987), p. 483.

Kottegoda, S.R. "Cheese, Wine and Isoniazid." *The Lancet,* (November 9, 1985), p. 1074.

Meydani, E.M. "Effects of Sucrose Polyester (SPE) on the Absorption of Dietary Vitamins A and E." Abstract, p. 697.

Griffin, M.J.J. and Morris, James S. "MAOI-like Reaction Associated with Cimetidine." *Drug Intelligence and Clinical Pharmacy,* (February, 1987), p. 219.

Randle, Ned W. "Food or Nutrient Effects on Drug Absorption: A Review." *Hospital Pharmacy,* (July 1987), pp. 694-697.

Zetin, Mark. "MAOI Reaction with Powdered Protein Dietary Supplement." *Journal of Clinical Psychiatry,* (December 1987), p. 499.

"Foods Interacting with MAOI Inhibitors." *The Medical Letter,* Vol. 31, Issue 785, (February 10, 1989), pp. 11-12.

Pagenkopf, Andrea and Mullen, Lisa. "Nutrition and the Elderly: Food-Drug Interactions." *Montguide (MT 8518),* Montana Cooperative Extension Service, Montana State University, Bozeman, MT.

Ling, Michael H. M. "An Overview on Food-Drug Interactions." *The Journal of Practising Pharmacists,* Vol. 6, No. 2, (Apr/Jun, 1988), pp. 6975.

Foye, William O. Principles Of Medicinal Chemistry. Lea and Febiger, Philadelphia, (1974).

Anderson, Karl E. "Influences of Diet and Nutrition on Clinical Pharmacokinetics." *Clinical Pharmacokinetics,* Vol. 14, (1988), pp. 325-246.

"Food and Drug Interactions." A brochure sponsored by the American Pharmaceutical Association; FDA; Food Marketing Institute; National Consumers League, Washington, D.C.

Stockley, Ivan H. "Drugs, foods and environmental chemical agents which can initiate antabuse-like reactions with alcohol." *Pharmacy International,* (January 1983), pp. 12-16.

"Drug Interactions with Monoamine Oxidase Inhibitors." *Drug Information Bulletin,* Vol. 22, No. 8, (Dec. 1988).

Cerrato, Paul L. "Drugs and Food: When the Dangers Increase." *RN,* (November 1988), pp. 65-67.

Schwinghammer, Terry L. and Giovannitti, Christine. "Guide to Important Food and Drug Considerations." *Nursing*, (August, 1988), pp. 40-41.

Sherman, David. "Drug Therapy Can Affect Diet." *Contemporary Long-Term Care,* (September 1990), pp. 72-74.

"Sulfasalazine Inhibits Folate Absorption." *Nutritional Reviews,* Vol. 46, No. 9, (September 1988), pp. 320-322.

Dowling, Teresa P. "The Use of Vitamins." *American Druggist,* (August, 1983), pp. 59-66.

Schein, Jeff. "Some Foods and Drugs Don't Mix." *Consumers' Research,* (March 1987), pp. 33-37.

"Food and Drug Interactions." *Consult,* Computerized literature search with abstracts from Merck, Sharp & Dohme.

"Food Terminology: What It Says Is Not Always What It Is." *U.S. Pharmacist,* (February 1980), p. 33.

Hopkins, Harold. "The GRAS List Revisited." *FDA Consumer,* (May, 1978).

"Food for Thought: A Basic Guide to Nutrition." *The Apothecary,* (November/December 1980), pp. 8-16.

Gibson, Anne and Clancy, R. "Management of chronic idiopathic urticaria by the identification and exclusion of dietary factors." *Clinical Allergy,* Vol. 10, No. 6, (November 1980), pp. 699-704.

Doeglas, H.M.G. "Reactions to aspirin and food additives in patients with chronic urticaria, including the physical urticarias." *British Journal of Dermatology,* Vol. 93, (1975), pp. 135-143.

Ortolani, C.; Pastorello, E. and Zanussi, C. "Prophylaxis of adverse reactions to foods: A double-blind study of oral sodium cromoglycate for the prophylaxis of adverse reactions to foods and additives." *Annals of Allergy,* Vol. 50, (February, 1983), pp. 105-109.

Guary, David R. P. "Drug-Nutrient Interactions." *Canadian Pharmacy Journal,* (July 1985), pp. 336-339.

"Alcohol in Foods." Guidelines for Antabuse (Disulfiram) Users, Ayerst Laboratories, (January 1981), pp. 8-11.

Pagliaro, Louis A. and Locock, Robert A. "Aspartame." *Revue Pharmaceutique Canadienne,* (March 1986), pp. 121-123.

"Foods potentially harmful to patients taking MAO Inhibitors." *The Medical Letter,* Vol. 18, No. 7, (March 26, 1976), p. 32.

"Megavitamin Therapy and Adverse Effects." *Hospital Formulary,* (August, 1979), p. 781.

Mesmer, Roger E. "Don't Mix Miso with MAOIs." *Journal of the American Medical Association,* Vol. 258, No. 24, (Dec. 25, 1987), p. 3515.

Jones, B.D. and Runikis, A.M. "Interaction of Ginseng with Phenelzine." *Journal of Clinical Psychopharmacology,* Vol. 7., No. 3, (June 1987), pp. 201-202.

Vesell, Elliot S. "Complex effects of diet on drug disposition." *Clinical Pharmacology and Therapeutics,* Vol. 36, No. 3, (Sept. 1984), pp. 285-296.

Mayo Clinic Diet Manual—A Handbook of Dietary Practices. W.B. Saunders Co., Philadelphia, (1981), pp. 123-125.

Pierpaoli, Paul G. "Drug Therapy and Diet." *Drug Intelligence and Clinical Pharmacy,* Vol. 6, (March 1972), pp. 89-99.

"Antihypertensive Drugs." Meyler's Side Effects Of Drugs (9th ed.), (1980).

Gallo, Nick. "When food and drugs clash." *Better Homes and Gardens,* (March 1988), pp. 87-88.

Noakes, T.D. "Prudent diet supplies adequate pyridoxine." *SAMJ,* Vol. 70, (August 16, 1986), p. 190.

Rogers, George A. "Flavors altered by lithium." *American Journal of Psychiatry,* Vol. 138, No. 2, (February 1981), p. 261.

Willoughby, J.M.T. "Drug-Induced Abnormalities of Taste Sensation." *Adverse Drug Reaction Bulletin,* Adverse Drug Reaction Research Unit, Shotley Bridge General Hospital, Consett, Co. Durham, DH8 ONB. (June, 1983).

Jefferson, James W. "Lithium tremor and caffeine intake: two cases of drinking less and shaking more." *Journal of Clinical Psychiatry*, Vol. 49, No. 2, (February 1988), pp. 72-73.

"Lithium Carbonate Interactions." Hansten's Drug Interactions (5th ed.), (1985), p. 413.

Facts and Comparisons. Facts and Comparison, Inc., Division of J. B. Lippincott Company, St. Louis, Mo., (1991).

Roine, Risto, et. al. "Aspirin Increases Blood Alcohol Concentrations in Humans After Ingestion of Ethanol." *Journal of the American Medical Association,* Vol. 264, No. 18, (November 14, 1990), pp. 2406-2408.

Lane, Elizabeth A.; Guthrie, Sally; and Linnoila, Markku. "Effects of Ethanol on Drug Metabolite Pharmacokinetics." *Clinical Pharmacokinetics,* Vol. 10, (1985), pp. 228-247.

Pinto, J. T. "The Pharmacokinetic and Pharmacodynamic Interactions of Foods and Drugs." *Topics in Clinical Nutrition,* Vol. 6, No. 3, (1991), pp. 14-33.

Herbert, Victor; Subak-Sharpe, Genell J.; and Hammock, Delia A. The Mount Sinai School of Medicine Complete Book of Nutrition. St. Martin's Press, New York, (1990), pp. 335-340.

Dawson, G.W.; Jue, S.G.; and Brogden, R.N. "Alprazolam: A Review of Its Pharmacodynamic Properties and Efficacy in the Treatment of Anxiety and Depression." Abstract citing *Drugs,* Vol. 25, (1984), pp. 132-147.

Terrell, Howard B. "Behavioral Dyscontrol Associated with Combined Use of Alprazolam and Ethanol" (letter). *American Journal of Psychiatry,* Vol. 145, No. 10, (October,1988), pp. 1313.

Linnoila, M; et. al. "Effects of Single Doses of Alprazolam and Diazepam, Alone and in Combination with Ethanol, on Psychomotor and Cognitive Performance and on Automonic Nervous System Reactivity in Health Volunteers." Abstract citing *European Journal of Clinical Pharmacology*, Vol. 39, (1990), pp. 21-28.

Kaplan, Gary B.; et. al. "Separate and Combined Effects of Caffeine and Alprazolam on Motor Activity and Benzodiazepine receptor Binding in Vivo." Abstract citing *Psychopharmacology,* Vol. 101, (1990), pp. 539-544.

Scavone, J.; Greenblatt, D; and Shader, R. "Alprazolam Kinetic Following Sublingual and Oral Administration." Abstract citing *Journal of Clinical Psychopharmacology*, Vol. 7, No. 5, (October 1987), pp. 332-334.

Garzone, Pamela D.; and Kroboth, Patricia D. "Pharmacokinetics of the Newer Benzodiazepines." Abstract citing *Clinical Pharmacokinetics*, Vol. 16, (1989), pp. 337-364.

Eller, Mark G. and Della-Coletta, Andrew A. "Absence of Effect of food on Alprazolam Absorption from Sustained Release Tablets." Abstract citing *Biopharmaceutics and Drug Disposition*, Vol. 11, (1990), pp. 31-37.

Cohen, Michael R. "The Benzodiazepines—A Review." *Hospital Pharmacy*, Vol. 20, No. 10, (October, 1985), pp. 767-769.

Ballinger, Brian R. "Hypnotics and Anxiolytics." *British Medical Journal*, Vol. 300, (February 17, 1990), pp. 456-458.

Goa, Karen; and Ward, Alan. "Buspirone: A Preliminary Review of Its Pharmacological Properties and Therapeutic Efficacy as an Anxiolytic." Abstract citing *Drugs*, Vol. 32, (1986), pp. 114-129.

Olkkola, K.T. and Neuvonen, P.J. "Effect of Food on the Antidotal Efficacy of Oral Activated Charcoal in Man." Abstract citing *Journal of Toxicology and Clinical Toxicology*, Vol. 23, No. 6, (1985), p. 447.

Harder, Sebastian; Fuhr, Uwe; and Staib, A. Horst. "Ciprofloxacin-Caffeine: A Drug Interaction Established Using In Vivo and In Vitro Investigations." Abstract citing *The American Journal of Medicine*, Vol. 87, Suppl. 5a, (November 30, 1989), pp. 89s-91s.

Polk, Ron E. "Drug-Drug Interactions with Ciprofloxacin and Other Fluoroquinolones." Abstract citing *The American Journal of Medicine*, Vol. 87, Suppl. 5a, (November 30, 1989), pp. 76s-81s.

Staib, A.H., et. al. "Interaction Between Quinolones and Caffeine." Abstract citing *Drugs*, Vol. 34, Suppl. 1, (1987), pp. 170-174.

Frost, R., et. al. "Ciprofloxacin Pharmacokinetics After a Standard or High-Fat/High-Calcium Breakfast." Abstract citing *Journal of Clinical Pharmacology*, Vol. 29, (1989), pp. 953-955.

Kara, M., et. al. "Clinical and Chemical Interactions Between Iron Preparations and Ciprofloxacin." Abstract citing *British Journal of Clinical Pharmacology*, Vol. 31, (1991), pp. 257-261.

Campbell, Norman and Hasinoff, Brian B. "Iron Supplements: A Common Cause of Drug Interactions." Abstract citing *British Journal of Clinical Pharmacology*, Vol. 31, (1991), pp. 251-255.

Peters II, Mark D.; Davis, Sharon K.; Austin, Linda S. "Clomipramine: An Antiobsessional Tricyclic Antidepressant." Abstract citing *Clinical Pharmacy*, Vol. 9, No. 3, (March 1990), pp. 165-178.

Joeres, Rolf and Richter, Ernst. "Mexiletine and Caffeine Clearance" (letter). *New England Journal of Medicine*, Vol. 317, No. 2, (July, 1987), p. 117.

Naranjo, Claudio A., et. al. "Gluoxetine Differentially Alters Alcohol Intake and Other Consummatory Behaviors in Problem Drinkers." Abstract citing *Clinical Pharmacology and Therapeutics*, Vol. 47, No. 4, (April, 1990), pp. 490-498.

Ciraulo, Domenic A. and Shader, Richard I. "Fluoxetine Drug—Drug Interactions II." Abstract citing *Journal of Clinical Psychopharmacology,* Vol. 10, No. 3, (June, 1990), pp. 213-217.

Johnson, A., et. al. "The Effect of Spontaneous Changes in Urinary pH on Mexiletine Plasma Concentrations and Excretion During Chronic Administration to Health Volunteers." Abstract citing *British Journal of Clinical Pharmacology,* Vol. 8, (1979), pp. 349-352.

Chew, C.Y.C.; Collett, J.; and Singh, B.N. "Mexiletine: A Review of Its Pharmacological Properties and Therapeutic Efficacy in Arrhythmias." Abstract citing *Drugs,* Vol. 17, (1979), pp. 161-181.

Mitchell, B.G.; et. al. "Mexiletine Disposition: Individual Variations in Response to Urine Acidification and Alkalinisation." Abstract citing *British Journal of Clinical Pharmacology,* Vol. 16, (1983), pp. 281-284.

Johnston, A., et. al. "Mexiletine Elimination: Influence of Urinary pH and Volume." Abstract citing *British Journal of Pharmacology,* Vol. 72, (1981), p. 135p.

Schrader, Bruce J. and Bauman, Jerry L. "Mexiletine: A New Type I Antiarrhythmic Agent." Abstract citing *Drug Intelligence and Clinical Pharmacy,* Vol. 20, No. 4, (April, 1986), pp. 255-260.

Campbell, Ronald. "Mexiletine." Abstract citing *New England Journal of Medicine,* Vol. 316, No. 1, (January 1, 1987), pp. 29-34.

Goldstein, Ellie. "Norfloxacin: first of the New Oral Fluoroquinolone Antibacterials." Abstract citing *Hospital Formulary,* Vol. 22, (May, 1987), pp. 462-477.

Holmes, B.; Brogden, R.N.; and Richards, D.M. "Norfloxacin: A Review of Its Antibacterial Activity, Pharmacokinetic Properties, and Therapeutic Use." Abstract citing *Drugs,* Vol. 30, (1985), pp. 482-513.

Monk, Jon P. and Campoli-Richards, Deborah M. "Ofloxacin: A Review of Its Antibacterial Activity, Pharmacokinetic Properties and Therapeutic Use." Abstract citing *Drugs*, Vol. 33, (1987), pp. 346-391.

Pilbrant, A. and Cederberg, C. "Development of an Oral Formulation of Omeprazole." Abstract citing *Scandinavian Journal of Gastroenterology*, Vol. 20, Suppl. 108, (1985), pp. 113-120.

Rohss, K., et. al. "Bioavailability of Omeprazol Given in Conjunction with Food." Abstract citing *Acta Pharmacologica et Toxicologica,* Vol. 59, Suppl. V, (1986), p. 85.

Shmueli, U. and Record, C.O. "Adverse Effects of Ulcer-Healing Drugs." Abstract citing *Adverse Drug Reaction Bulletin,* No. 147, (April, 1991), pp. 552-555.

Kando, Judith C. and Kalunian, Douglas A. "Focus on Selegiline: A Selective Monoamine Oxidase Type B Inhibitor." Abstract citing *Hospital Formulary,* Vol. 25, No. 8, (August, 1990), pp. 849, ff.

Sunter, J.P.; Bal, T.S.; and Cowan, W.K. "Three Cases of Fatal Triazolam Poisoning." Abstract citing *British Medical Journal,* Vol. 297, (September 17, 1988), p. 719.

O'Dowd, J.J.; Spragg, P.P.; and Routledge, P.A. "Fatal Triazolam Poisoning." Abstract citing *British Medical Journal,* Vol. 297, (October 22, 1988), p. 1048.

Lane, Elizabeth A.; Guthrie, Sally; and Linnoila, Markku. "Effects of Ethanol on Drug and Metabolite Pharmacokinetics." Abstract citing *Clinical Pharmacokinetics,* Vol. 10, (1985), pp. 228-247.

Lee, Connie R.; McKenzie, Constance A.; and Mantooth, Rusty. "Food and Drug Interactions." *U.S. Pharmacist,* (May, 1991), pp. 44 ff.

Flodin, N. W. "Micronutrient Supplements: Toxicity and Drug Interactions." *Progress in Good and Nutrition Science,* Vol. 14, (1990), pp. 277-331.

Messner, Roberta L. and Gardner, Sylvia S. "Drug Interactions We all Overlook." *RN,* Vol. 56, No. 1, (January 1993), pp. 50 ff.

Serpa, Maria D. and McGreevy, M. Joseph, "Drug Complications Case & Comment." *Patient Care,* Vol. 26, No. 11, (July 15, 1992), p. 278.

Katcher, Brian S. "Food and Drugs that Don't Mix."

"Nicotine Gum Users: Watch What You Drink." *Science News,* Vol. 138, p. 220.

Molyneux, ME, et al., "Efficacy of Quinine for Falciparum Malaria According to Previous Chloroquine Exposure." *The Lancet,* Vol. 337, (June 8, 1991), pp. 1379 ff.

Bailey, David G., et al., "Interaction of Citrus Juices with Felodipine and Nifedipine." *The Lancet,* Vol. 337, (February 2, 1991), pp. 268 ff.

Alderman, Michael, et al., "Addressing Multiple Risks in Hypertension Therapy." *Patient Care,* Vol. 28, No. 14, (September 15, 1994), pp. 64 ff.

Sorgel, Fritz, et al., "Comparative Pharmacokinetics of Ciprofloxacin and Temafloxacin in Humans: A Review," *The American Journal of Medicine,* Vol. 91, (December 30, 1991), pp. 6A-51S ff.

Gauvin, David V.; Peirce, Jessica M.; and Holloway, Frank A. "Perceptual Masking of the Chlordiazepoxide Discriminative Cue by both Caffeine and Buspirone." *Pharmacology, Biochemistry and Behavior,* Vol. 47, (January 1994), pp. 153 ff.

Stanwood, Les, "The Double Whammy of Alchol and Drugs." *Current Health,* (October 1990), pp. 26 ff.

Forster, Lorna Earl; Pollow, Rachel; and Stoller, Eleanor P., "Alcohol Use and Potential Risk for Alcohol-related Adverse Drug Reactions among Community-based Elderly." *Journal of Community Health,* Vol. 18, No. 4, (August 1993), pp. 225.

Smith, H.T., et al., "Pharmacokinetics of Fluvastatin and Specific Drug Interactions." *The American Journal of Hypertension,* Vol. 6, No. 11, (November 1993), pp. 375S ff.

Sides, Gregory D, et al., "Pharmacokinetics of Dirithromycin." *Journal of Antimicrobial Chemotherapy,* Vol. 31, (March 1993), pp. 65 ff.

Joshi, M.V., et al., "Food Reduces Isoniazid Bioavailability in Normal Volunteers." *Journal of Association of Physicians of India,* Vol., 39, No. 6, (June 1991), pp. 470 ff.

Schein, Jeffrey R. "Food and Drugs that Don't Mix." *Consumer's Digest,* Vol. 29, No. 4, (July/August 1990), pp. 55 ff.

Winter, Ruth, "Which Pain Relievers Work Best?" *Consumers Digest,* Vol. 33, No. 5, (September/October 1994), pp. 74 ff.

Schmidt, Elizabeth B. "Drug Interactions." *Harvard Health Letter,* Vol. 18, No. 3, (Jan 1993), pp. 4 ff.

Kuhn, Merrily "Drug Interactions and Their Nursing Implications." *Journal of the New York State Nurses Association,* Vol. 24, No. 2, (June 1993), pp. 10 ff.

Pappas, Nancy "Dangerous Liaisons: When Food and Drugs Don't Mix." Vol. 36, No. 16, (October 28, 1991).

"Drug Interactions—What Your Patient Needs to Know." *Nursing* 94, Vol. 24, No. 9, (September 1994), pp. 32M ff.

Chase, Sandra, "Antacids." *RN,* (August 1993), pp. 46 ff.

Cerrato, Paul L. "Vitamins and Minerals." *RN,* Vol. 56, No. 6, (June 1993), pp. 28 ff.

Rodman, Morton J. "Analgesics and Anti-Inflammatories." *RN,* Vol. 50, No. #1, (January 1993), pp. 54 ff.

Rodman, Morton J. "Asthma Medications." *RN,* Vol. 56, No. 4, (April 1993), pp. 40 ff.

McKee, R.H. and Scala, R.A., "Interactions: The Effects of Chemicals on each Other." *Toxic Substances Journal,* Vol. 13, No. 2, (April/June 1994), pp. 71 ff.

Cicalese, Gerard T. "Trichomoniasis and Alcohol Dependency." Vol. 32, No. 5, (May 1992), p. 27.

Rodman, Morton J. "Cough, Cold and Allergy Preparations." *RN,* Vol. 56, No. 2, (February 1993), pp. 38 ff.

Alkhawajah, A.M. and Eferakeya, A.E., "The Role of Pharmacists in Patients' Education on Medication." *Public Health,* Vol. 106, No. 3, (May 1992), pp. 231 ff.

Patierno, Steven R. "Role of Chemical Delivery Modes in Toxicological Studies." *Toxic Substances Journal,* Vol. 11, No. 2, (April/June 1991), pp. 111 ff.

Knodel, Leroy C. "Nonsedating Antihistamines and the Risk of Serious Cardiovascular Events." *Toxic Substances Journal,* Vol. 13, No. 1, (January/March 1994), pp. 65 ff.

Kehoe, William A. "Grape Fruit Juice-Drug Interactions." Pharmacist's Letter, Document #130405.

"Food/Drug Interactions Checklist." St. Francis Medical Center, Monroe, LA, (1997).

Andel, Micheline, "Antibiotic Food Interactions." Wellcome Trends in Hospital Pharmacy, (May 1991), p. 15.

INDEX

A

Acarbose **A:** 1
ACE Inhibitors **A:** 2
Acetaminophen **A:** 3-5
Acetazolamide **A:** 6, 7
Acid Beverages **A:** 38; **P:** 10
Acidic Foods **N:** 16
Adrenal Corticosteroids **A:** 8-10
Alcohol **A:** 3, 11-15, 17, 27, 42, 46, 47, 49, 55, 62, 67, 68, 71, 76, 80, 92, 93; **B:** 2, 10, 15, 22, 23, 26; **C:** 6, 19, 25, 26, 30, 38, 39, 42, 56, 58, 62, 63, 71, 79; **D:** 6, 19, 22, 23, 34, 37; **E:** 18; **F:** 8, 10, 15, 17, 21; **G:** 4, 5, 9, 11; **H:** 1, 3, 56, 11, 18, 25; **I:** 1, 3, 8, 16; **L:** 18; **M:** 1, 8, 14, 16, 32, 34, 45; **N:** 23, 24, 30, 28; **P:** 1, 14, 15, 25, 33, 43, 54, 55, 58, 61; **S:** 7, 8, 12, 15, 34; **T:** 30, 33, 36; **U:** 1; **V:** 1, 9, 11, 15; **W:** 1
Aldendronate **A:** 16
Alkaline Foods **A:** 87; **B:** 20; **E:** 9
Allopurinol **A:** 17
Almonds **B:** 20
Alprazolam **A:** 17, 19, 20
Aluminum **D:** 3; **T:** 3
Aluminum Hydroxide **A:** 20, 45
Amiloride **A:** 22
Amino Acids **A:** 50; **C:** 27, 64; **E:** 10; **I:** 25; K: 1; L: 4; **M:** 29; **N:** 10; **O:** 3; **P:** 2, 11, 45; **S:** 41; **T:** 4
Aminoglycosides **A:** 23-26
Amitriptyline **A:** 27-30
Amlodipine **C:** 8, 31
Ammonium Chloride **A:** 32, 33
Amoxicillin **A:** 34, 40
Amphetamine **A:** 35-37
Ampicillin **A:** 38, 39
Antacids **A:** 43-45; **B:** 1; **D:** 36
Anti-Angina Drugs **A:** 42, 46, 47
Anti-Arrhythmia Drugs **A:** 48
Anti-Inflammatory Drugs **A:** 74
Antibiotics **A:** 49-53

Anticholinergics **A:** 54
Anticoagulants **A:** 55-61
Anticonvulsants **A:** 62-67
Antihistamines **A:** 68-70
Antihypertensives **A:** 71-74
Antipsychotics **A:** 76-78
Antituberculars **A:** 79
Apples **D:** 13
Applesauce **I:** 9
Aspartame **D:** 24
Aspirin **A:** 80-90
Astemizole **A:** 91
Atabrine **A:** 92
Atenolol **A:** 93-95
Atovaquone **A:** 96
Atropine **A:** 97
Azithromycin **A:** 98
Azulfidine **A:** 99

B

Bacon **G:** 11
Baking Soda **B:** 1
Barbequed Foods **T:** 11
Barbiturates **B:** 2-9
Beans **P:** 35
Benzodiazepines **B:** 10-14
Beta Carotene **B:** 19
Beta-Blockers **B:** 15,16
Biguanides **B:** 17, 18
Bile Acid Sequestrants **B:** 19
Bisacodyl **B:** 20, 21
Bleomycin **V:** 8
Blood Pressure Medications **B:** 22
Bran **D:** 13; **Z:** 6
Bread **M:** 23; **Z:** 6
Broccoli **W:** 2
Brompheniramine **B:** 23
Bronchodilators **B:** 24, 25
Brussels Sprouts **A:** 4; **P:** 64; **T:** 27; **W:** 2
Buspirone **B:** 26, 27
Butter **G:** 11; **M:** 23

C

Cabbage **A:** 4; **P:** 64; **T:** 27
Caffeine **A:** 19, 48, 81; **B:** 11, 24; **C:** 1, 2, 21, 31, 45, 51,

66; **D:** 3, 21, 25, 26, 36; **E:** 11, 27; **F:** 5, 19; **G:** 3, 7; **H:** 4, 17; **I:** 10, 19, 20, 27; **K:** 2; **L:** 3, 11; **M:** 6, 27, 38, 41; **N:** 11, 31, 33, 34; **P:** 32; **S:** 9; **T:** 10; **U:** 2

Calcium **A:** 8, 21, 23, 51, 63, 94; **B:** 16, 21; **C:** 3-7, 12, 17, 27, 44, 52, 57, 72, 80; **D:** 3, 21, 26, 36; **E:** 11; **F:** 5, 19; **G:** 3, 7; **H:** 17; **I:** 10, 20, 27; **K:** 2; **L:** 3; **M:** 27, 41; **N:** 11, 33; **P:** 3, 11, 18, 24, 34, 45; **Q:** 9; **S:** 11, 25, 42; **T:** 3, 20, 29; **V:** 4, 20
Calcium Acetate **C:** 5
Calcium Carbimide **C:** 6
Calcium Carbonate **C:** 7
Calcium Channel Blockers **C:** 8
Canteloupe **P:** 35
Captopril **C:** 9
Carbamazepine **C:** 10, 11
Carbohydrates **A:** 5, 23; **B:** 25; **C:** 57; **D:** 13; **H:** 18; **N:** 11; **T:** 17, 18
Carbonated Beverages **A:** 38; **C:** 38, 61; **E:** 8; **F:** 12; **P:** 10
Cardiac Glycosides **C:** 12-16
Carotene **C:** 44, 57, 64; **M:** 24, 41; **N:** 11
Carrageenan **P:** 40
Carrots **P:** 64; **T:** 27
Caseinates **P:** 40
Cathartics **C:** 17
Cauliflower **P:** 64; **T:** 27
Cefaclor **C:** 18
Cefamandol **C:** 19, 22
Cefoperazone **C:** 19, 22
Cefotetan **C:** 19, 22
Cefuroxime **C:** 20
Cephalexin **C:** 23
Cephalosporins **C:** 18-20, 22, 23
Cephradine **C:** 23
Cereal **C:** 3, 15; **I:** 20
Charcoal **C:** 24
Charcoal-Broiled Food **B:** 3, 12; **P:** 36; **T:** 11; **W:** 3
Cheese **A:** 45; **S:** 10; **T:** 3
Chestnuts **B:** 20
Chloral Hydrate **C:** 25
Chloramphenicol **C:** 26-29
Chlordiazepoxide **C:** 30, 31
Chlorhexidine **C:** 32
Chloride **D:** 26; **S:** 18
Chlorine **F:** 19
Chloroquine **C:** 33-35
Chlorothiazide **C:** 36, 37
Chlorpheniramine **C:** 38

Chlorpromazine **C:** 39-41
Chlorpropamide **C:** 42
Chlortetracycline **C:** 43
Chocolate **C:** 3
Cholesterol **C:** 44, 57, 64, 65; **G:** 2; **M:** 24; **N:** 11; **O:** 4; **S:** 53; **Z:** 4
Cholestyramine **C:** 44
Cimetidine **C:** 45-49
Cinoxacin **C:** 50
Ciprofloxacin **C:** 51
Cisplatin **C:** 53; **V:** 8
Clarithromycin **C:** 54
Clays **I:** 20
Clindamycin **C:** 55
Clobazam **C:** 56
Clofibrate **C:** 57
Clomipramine **C:** 58
Clonidine **C:** 59
Cloxacillin **C:** 60, 61
Cocaine **C:** 62
Coconut Oil **P:** 40
Codeine **C:** 63
Coffee **A:** 48, 77; **B:** 11, 24; **C:** 21, 31, 45; **E:** 2; **F:** 11; **H:** 2; **I:** 18, 19; **M:** 6; **N:** 14, 16, 31, 34; **P:** 26, 32; **T:** 10; **V:** 13
Cola beverages **B:** 11; **C:** 21, 31, 45; **E:** 2; **I:** 19; **M:** 6; **N:** 16, 34; **P:** 32; **T:** 10
Colchicine **C:** 64
Colestipol **C:** 65
Contraceptives (oral) **C:** 66-69; **O:** 3-9
Cooking Oils **A:** 56
Copper **C:** 52, 70; **E:** 1; **M:** 2; **O:** 5; **P:** 5; **T:** 3
Corn Flakes **M:** 23
Corn Oil **P:** 40
Corticosteroids **C:** 71-73
Cortisol **C:** 74
Coumarin **C:** 75-77
Crackers **A:** 5
Cyclamates **L:** 9
Cyclophosphamide **C:** 78
Cycloserine **C:** 79-82
Cyclosporine **C:** 83, 84

D

Dairy Products **B:** 20; **C:** 52; **D:** 3, 21, 36; **E:** 9; **F:** 5; **H:** 17; **I:** 20; **T:** 3
Dapsone **D:** 1

Dates **A:** 5
Decongestants **N:** 8, 9; **S:** 54
Demeclocycline **D:** 2, 3
Depressants **C:** 21
Desipramine **D:** 4, 5
Diazepam **D:** 6-8
Dicloxacillin **D:** 9
Dicoumarol **D:** 10
Didanosine **D:** 11
Diet Medications **S:** 54
Digestive Enzymes **D:** 12
Digitalis **D:** 13-18
Digoxin **D:** 13-18
Diphenhydramine **D:** 19
Dirithromycin **D:** 20, 21
Disopyramide **D:** 22
Disulfiram **D:** 23-25
Diuretics **D:** 26-32; **F:** 19, 20; **S:** 18; **T:** 20-26, 34, 35
Doxyrubicin **D:** 33
Doxycycline **D:** 34-36
Dronabinol **D:** 37
DSS **D:** 38

E

EDTA **E:** 1
Eggs **I:** 20; **L:** 6
Egg Yolk **A:** 45
Electrolytes **C:** 17, 44, 57, 64; **D:** 26; **L:** 3, 14; **N:** 11
Enoxacin **E:** 2, 3
Enteric-Coated Medicines **E:** 4, 9
Ephedrine **E:** 5
Ergotamine **E:** 7
Erythromycin **E:** 8-12
Estrogens **E:** 13-16
Ethacrynic Acid **E:** 17
Ethchlorvynol **E:** 18
Etodolac **E:** 19

F

Famotidine **F:** 1
Fat **A:** 11; **B:** 21; **C:** 7, 27, 44, 57, 64, 65; **D:** 10, 14; **G:** 1, 2, 11, 13; **I:** 12; **L:** 3; **M:** 3, 15, 24, 44; **N:** 11, 19; **P:** 3, 24; **Q:** 3; **R:** 2; **S:** 11, 20, 26
Fatty Acids **N:** 11
Felodipine **C:** 8; **F:** 2

Ferrous Sulfate **F:** 3
Fiber **C:** 4, 15; **D:** 13; **S:** 21; **V:** 14
5-Fluorouracil **F:** 7
Flecanide **F:** 4
Fluoride **A:** 44; **F:** 5
Fluoroquinolones **F:** 6
Fluoxetine **F:** 8, 9
Fluphenazine **F:** 11; **N:** 14
Flurazepam **F:** 10
Fluvastatin **F:** 12
Fluvoxamine **F:** 14
Folic Acid **A:** 11, 53, 64, 79, 83, 99; **B:** 4; **C:** 27, 44, 67, 81; **E:** 11, 13; **F:** 15; **I:** 28; **K:** 1; **M:** 25; **N:** 4, 11; **O:** 6; **P:** 3, 11, 13, 19, 24, 35, 38, 45, 51, 65; **S:** 1, 37; **T:** 5, 34, 40
Food **A:** 1, 5, 9, 12, 16, 20, 34, 39, 40, 41, 52, 54, 72, 82, 91, 95, 96, 98; **B:** 13, 21, 27; **C:** 5, 9, 10, 18, 24, 27, 32, 36, 40, 43, 46, 50, 54, 55, 57, 60, 83; **D:** 2, 8, 9-13, 20, 35 ; **E:** 3, 4; **F:** 1, 12, 13, 16, 20; **G:** 6, 11; **H:** 12, 15; **I:** 2, 11, 29, 32, 37, 38; **L:** 1, 2, 4, 5, 8, 12, 16, 19; **M:** 17, 23, 28, 33, 35, 39, 42, 43; **N:** 1, 19, 25, 29, 32, 35, 38; **O:** 1, 2, 10, 11, 14; **P:** 6, 12, 20, 28, 37, 44, 46, 50, 57, 59, 62; **Q:** 4; **R:** 1, 3; **S:** 6, 13, 17, 19, 24, 26, 27, 32, 33, 36, 40, 44, 52; **T:** 1, 6, 12, 13, 28, 32; **V:** 2, 12, 14; **Z:** 1, 2, 3, 5
Fosinopril **F:** 16
Fructose **B:** 8
Fruit **A:** 38; **E:** 8
Fruit Juices **C:** 61; **E:** 8; **I:** 21; **N:** 16, 31; **P:** 10
Furazolidone **F:** 17, 18
Furosemide **F:** 19, 20
Furoxone **F:** 21

G

Ganciclovir **G:** 1
Gemfibrozil **G:** 2
Gensing **P:** 16
Gentamicin **G:** 3
Glibenclamide **G:** 4
Glipizide **G:** 5, 6
Glucocorticoids **G:** 7, 8
Glucose **B:** 8, 17, 21; **L:** 3; **O:** 7; **P:** 24
Glutethimide **G:** 9, 10
Glycyrrihizic Acid **H:** 7
Grape Fruit Juice **A:** 31; **C:** 1, 8, 84; **E:** 14; **F:** 2; **M:** 40; **N:** 15, 20, 22; **T:** 2, 37; **V:** 5

Griseofulvin G: 11-13
Guanethidine G: 14

H

Haloperidol **H:** 2; **N:** 14
Heart Medications **H:** 3, 4
Heparin **H:** 5
Herbal Teas **A:** 85
High Blood Pressure Medications **H:** 6-10
Histamine **I:** 31
H2 Blockers **H:** 1
Hydantoins **H:** 11
Hydralazine **H:** 12-14
Hydrochlorothiazide **H:** 15, 16
Hydrocortisone **H:** 17
Hypoglycemics **H:** 18-20

I

Ibuprofen **I:** 1, 2
Imipramine **I:** 3-6
Indinavir **I:** 7
Indomethacin **I:** 8-15
Ink Caps Fungus **A:** 13
Insulin **I:** 16-18
Iron **A:** 44, 86; **B:** 19; **C:** 28, 44, 47, 52, 57, 70; **D:** 3, 12, 36; **E:** 1; **F:** 3, 6; **G:** 2; **I:** 13, 19-23; **M:** 2, 27; **N:** 7, 11, 33; **O:** 5; **P:** 7, 11; **S:** 4, 14; **T:** 3; **V:** 6, 18; **W:** 6
Isocarboxazid **I:** 24
Isoniazid **I:** 25-34
Isotretinoin **I:** 35, 36
Isradipine **I:** 37
Itraconazole **I:** 38

J

Japanese Food **W:** 8
Jellies **A:** 5
Juices **A:** 38

K

Kale **P:** 64; **T:** 27

Kanamycin **K:** 1-4
Kaolin **C:** 55

L

Labetalol **L:** 1
Lactose **M:** 24; **N:** 11
Lansoprazole **L:** 2
Laxatives **L:** 3; **M:** 27
Legumes **C:** 3
Levodopa **L:** 4-7
Licorice **A:** 73; **C:** 13; **D:** 15, 28; **H:** 7; **T:** 21
Lincomycin **L:** 8-10
Lipids **B:** 19; **C:** 44, 65; **L:** 3; **M:** 41
Lithium **L:** 11-15
Liver **A:** 45; **D:** 29; **P:** 35
Lomefloxacin **L:** 16
Loratadine **L:** 17
Lorazepam **L:** 18
Lovastatin **L:** 19

M

Magnesium **A:** 11, 23, 53; **C:** 14, 27, 52, 53, 72, 80; **D:** 3, 16, 26, 36; **E:** 1, 11, 17; **F:** 19; **G:** 3; **I:** 27; **K:** 2; **M:** 1, 11, 27; **N:** 11, 33; **P:** 3, 11, 23, 45; **Q:** 9; **S:** 47; **T:** 3, 22, 29; **V:** 6; **W:** 6
Manganese **C:** 52, 70; **O:** 8
Mannitol **M:** 3
Margarine **G:** 11
Marijuana **M:** 8; **T:** 19
Meat **A:** 45; **D:** 29; **L:** 6; **T:** 3, 11
Mecamylamine **M:** 9, 10
Mefenamic Acid **M:** 11
Meperidine **M:** 12, 13
Meprobamate **M:** 14
Metamucil **M:** 15
Metformin **M:** 16, 17
Methadone **M:** 18
Methamphetamine **M:** 19, 20
Methenamine **M:** 21, 22
Methionine **A:** 11
Methotrexate **M:** 23-26
Methylcellulose **M:** 27
Methyldopa **M:** 28-31
Metoclopramide **M:** 32
Metoprolol **M:** 33

Metronidazole **M:** 34, 35
Mexiletine **M:** 36-39
Midazolam **M:** 40
Milk **A:** 45, 87; **B:** 20; **C:** 12, 52; **D:** 3, 21, 36; **E:** 9; **F:** 3; **I:** 20; **M:** 23; **P:** 48; **T:** 3, 31
Mineral Oil **M:** 41
Minerals **A:** 21; **C:** 17, 52; **N:** 21; **P:** 24, 41; **T:** 3; **Z:** 6
Misoprostol **M:** 42
Monoamine Oxidase Inhibitors (MAOIs) **M:** 4-7
Monosodium Glutamate (MSG) **D:** 30; **M:** 5; **P:** 39
Moricizine **M:** 43
Morphine **M:** 44
Moxalactam **C:** 22; **M:** 45, 46

N

Nafcillin **N:** 1
Nalidixic Acid **N:** 1, 2
Narcotics **N:** 4-7
Neomycin **N:** 10-13
Neuroleptic Agents **N:** 14
Niacin **I:** 33; **S:** 39
Nicardipine **N:** 15
Nicotinamide **O:** 9
Nicotine (gum) **N:** 16-18; **T:** 19
Nifedipine **C:** 8; **N:** 19-21
Nimodipine **C:** 8; **N:** 22
Nitrates **N:** 23
Nitrofurantoin **N:** 24-27
Nitrogen **A:** 11; **C:** 64
Nitroglycerin **N:** 28
Nizatidine **N:** 29
NonSteroidal Anti-Inflammatory Drugs (NSAIDs) **A:** 75; **N:** 30-32
Norfloxacin **N:** 33-35
Nortriptyline **N:** 36, 37
Novobiocin **N:** 38
Nutrients **C:** 44
Nuts **C:** 3; **P:** 35

O

Oflaxacin **O:** 1
Ondansetron **O:** 2
Onions **W:** 7
Oranges **P:** 35

Oxacillin **O:** 10
Oxalic Acid **C:** 3
Oxaprozin **O:** 11
Oxyphenbutazone **O:** 12, 13
Oxytetracycline **O:** 14

P

Pain Medications **P:** 1
Para-amino Benzoic Acid (PABA) **D:** 1; **M:** 26; **P:** 66
Para-Aminosalicylic Acid **P:** 2-4
Peaches **P:** 64; **T:** 27
Peanuts **A:** 45
Pears **D:** 13; **P:** 64; **T:** 27
Pectin **A:** 5; **C:** 55; **D:** 13; **L:** 10
Penicillamine **P:** 5-9
Penicillin **P:** 10-12
Pentamidine **P:** 13
Pentazocine **P:** 14
Pentobarbital **P:** 15
Phenelzine **P:** 16, 17
Phenobarbital **P:** 18-23
Phenolphthalein **P:** 24
Phenothiazines **P:** 25-27
Phenylbutazone **P:** 28-31
Phenylpropanolamine **P:** 32
Phenytoin **P:** 33-42
Phosphate **C:** 53; **I:** 14
Phosphorus **A:** 21, 44, 45; **M:** 41
Phytic Acid **C:** 3
Piroxicam **P:** 43, 44
Polymixin **P:** 45
Pork **G:** 11
Potassium **A:** 2, 22, 23, 53, 88; **B:** 21; **C:** 17, 37, 53, 64, 72; **D:** 17, 26, 27, 31; **E:** 17; **F:** 19; **G:** 3, 8; **H:** 16; **L:** 3, 14; **M:** 41; **N:** 11; **P:** 11, 24, 46-49; **S:** 11, 22; **T:** 7, 23, 29, 35
Pravastatin **P:** 50
Pressor Amines **F:** 18; **I:** 24; **M:** 4; **P:** 56; **S:** 54
Primidone **P:** 51
Probenecid **P:** 52, 53
Procainamide **P:** 54
Procarbazine **P:** 55, 56
Propantheline **P:** 57
Propoxyphene **P:** 58-60
Propranolol **P:** 61-63
Propylthiouracil **P:** 64

Protein **A:** 43; **B:** 7, 25; **C:** 27; **D:** 14; **I:** 12; **L:** 4, 6; **M:** 28, 44; **P:** 63; **S:** 20; **T:** 17, 18; **Z:** 6
Prune Juice **C:** 15
Pyrimethamine **P:** 65, 66

Q

Quinacrine **Q:** 1, 2
Quinapril **Q:** 3
Quinidine **Q:** 4-6
Quinine **C:** 35; **Q:** 7, 8
Quinolones **Q:** 9

R

Ramipril **R:** 1
Rctinol **V:** 8
Rifabutin **R:** 2
Rifampin **R:** 3
Rutabagas **P:** 64; **T:** 27

S

Salicylates **S:** 1-5
Salt **A:** 74; **E:** 15; **G:** 14; **H:** 8, 13; **I:** 15; **L:** 15; **M:** 30; **V:** 3
Salt Substitutes **D:** 31; **P:** 47
Saquinavir **S:** 6
Secobarbital **S:** 7
Sedatives **S:** 8
Selegiline **S:** 9, 10
Senna **S:** 11
Serotonin Reuptake Inhibitors **S:** 12
Sertraline **S:** 13
Silicone **A:** 56; **W:** 4
Simethicone **S:** 14
Sleeping Pills **S:** 15
Smoking **B:** 14; **C:** 2, 48; **F:** 4, 14; **H:** 9; **I:** 17; **P:** 60
Sodas **P:** 10
Sodium **A:** 9, 74, 75; **B:** 1; **C:** 59, 64, 73; **D:** 26, 27; **E:** 15; **F:** 19; **G:** 14; **H:** 8, 13; **I:** 15; **L:** 15; **M:** 30; **N:** 11; **P:** 8, 31; **S:** 16, 23, 28; **T:** 24; **V:** 3
Sodium Polystyrene **S:** 16
Sotalol **S:** 17
Soy Beans **P:** 64; **T:** 27

Soy Meal **W:** 8
Spinach **C:** 3; **P:** 64; **T:** 27; **W:** 2
Spironolactone **S:** 18-23
Starches **I:** 20; **P:** 40
Stavudine **S:** 24
Steroids **A:** 41; **S:** 25-29
Stool Softeners **S:** 53
Streptomycin **S:** 30, 31
Sucrose **B:** 8; **N:** 11
Sugar **A:** 89; **B:** 8; **C:** 44, 57, 64; **H:** 18; **M:** 23; **N:** 11; **P:** 24
Sucralfate **S:** 32
Sulfa Drugs **S:** 33-50
Sulfadiazine **S:** 36
Sulfasalazine **S:** 37
Sulfathiazole **S:** 38
Sulfinpyrazone **S:** 39
Sulfisoxazole **S:** 40
Sulfonamides **S:** 41-50
Sulfonylureas **S:** 51
Sumatriptan **S:** 52
Surfactants **D:** 38; **S:** 53
Sweet Clover **A:** 85
Sympathomimetics **S:** 54
Syrups **A:** 38; **E:** 8; **P:** 10

T

Tacrine **T:** 1
Tannic Acids **V:** 13
Tea **A:** 48, 77; **B:** 11, 24; **C:** 21, 31, 45; **E:** 2; **F:** 11; **H:** 2; **M:** 6; **N:** 14, 16, 31, 34 ; **I:** 19; **P:** 26, 32; **T:** 10; **V:** 13
Terfenadine **T:** 2
Tetracycline **T:** 3-9
Theophylline **T:** 10-19
Thiazides **T:** 20-26
Thyroid **T:** 27
Thyroxine **T:** 27
Ticlopidine **T:** 28
Tobacco **T:** 19
Tolazamide **T:** 30
Tolbutamide **T:** 30
Tolmetin **T:** 31, 32
Tobramycin **T:** 29
Tomatoes **E:** 8; **P:** 10
Tonic Water **C:** 35
Tonka Bean **A:** 85

Tranquilizers **T:** 33
Triamterene **T:** 34, 35
Triazolam **T:** 36, 37
Tricyclics **T:** 38, 39
Triglycerides **C:** 44, 57; **N:** 11; **O:** 4
Trimethoprim **T:** 40
l-Tryptophan **F:** 9; **M:** 7
Turnips **P:** 64; **T:** 27
Tyramine **C:** 49; **F:** 18; **H:** 10; **I:** 24, 30; **M:** 4; **P:** 17, 56; **S:** 54

U

Ulcer Medications **U:** 1, 2
Urates **A:** 17; **D:** 29; **P:** 53
Urinary Acidifiers **A:** 6, 24, 28, 32, 35, 69, 84, 97; **B:** 5; **C:** 33, 75; **D:** 4, 7; **E:** 5; **I:** 4; **M:** 9, 12, 19, 22, 36; **N:** 3, 5, 8, 17, 26, 36; **O:** 12; **P:** 21, 27, 29; **Q:** 1, 5, 7; **S:** 2, 3, 31, 35, 38, 45; **T:** 15, 38; **V:** 16; **W:** 5
Urinary Alkalinizers **A:** 7, 25, 29, 33, 36, 70; **B:** 6; **C:** 34, 75; **D:** 5; **E:** 6; **I:** 5; **K:** 3; **L:** 13; **M:** 10, 13, 20, 21, 37; **N:** 2, 6, 9, 17, 27, 37; **O:** 13; **P:** 22, 30; **Q:** 2, 6, 8; **S:** 3, 46; **T:** 16, 39; **V:** 17

V

Valproic Acid **V:** 1, 2
Vanilla Pudding **P:** 40
Vasodilators **V:** 3
Vegetables **A:** 4, 61; **B:** 20; **E:** 8, 9; **P:** 10, 35; **T:** 3, 14; **W:** 2
Verapamil **V:** 4-7
Vinblastine **V:** 8
Vitamin A **A:** 14, 26, 44; **B:** 19; **C:** 44, 57, 65, 68, 78; **D:** 26, 38; **G:** 2; **I:** 35; **M:** 15, 41; **N:** 11; **S:** 29, 53; **T:** 8; **V:** 9, 10, 21
Vitamin B **A:** 57, 79
Vitamin B_1 **A:** 11, 44; **C:** 16; **D:** 32; **F:** 7; 19; **O:** 9; **V:** 8, 11-13
Vitamin B_2 **C:** 41; **D:** 33; **I:** 6; **O:** 9; **P:** 52; **T:** 9; **V:** 14
Vitamin B_3 **A:** 79
Vitamin B_6 **A:** 53, 79; **C:** 27, 67, 72, 81; **E:** 11, 16; **H:** 14; **I:** 33; **K:** 4; **L:** 7; **N:** 12; **O:** 9; **P:** 9, 11, 23, 42, 45; **S:** 48; **T:** 9; **V:** 8
Vitamin B_{12} **A:** 11, 53, 78; **B:** 9, 18, 19; **C:** 27, 44, 57, 64, 80;

	E: 11; **G:** 2; **H:** 20; **I:** 27; **K:** 2; **M:** 24, 31; **N:** 11; **O:** 9; **P:** 3, 11, 23, 41, 45, 49, 51; **S:** 47; **T:** 9; **V:** 19
Vitamin C	**A:** 30, 37, 58, 90; **C:** 69, 72, 74; **E:** 16; **F:** 11; **I:** 21; **N:** 7; **O:** 9; **P:** 41; **S:** 5, 49; **T:** 9; **V:** 16-19; **W:** 9
Vitamin D	**A:** 10, 44, 65; **B:** 9, 19; **C:** 11, 44, 57, 64, 65, 72; **D:** 18; **G:** 2, 7, 10; **I:** 36; **M:** 15, 41; **N:** 11; **P:** 23, 24, 41; **T:** 25; **V:** 7, 20, 21
Vitamin E	**A:** 59; **B:** 19; **C:** 44, 57, 65; **G:** 2; **I:** 22; **M:** 15, 41; **V:** 8, 21; **W:** 10
Vitamin K	**A:** 53, 60, 66; **B:** 19; **C:** 29, 44, 57, 65, 77, 82; **G:** 2; **I:** 34; **M:** 41, 46; **N:** 11, 13; **P:** 4, 11, 23, 41; **S:** 50; **T:** 9; **V:** 10, 21; **W:** 11
Vitamins	**A:** 21; **C:** 17, 27, 44, 57, 64, 65, 72; **G:** 2; **L:** 3; **N:** 11; **O:** 9; **P:** 3, 41

W

Warfarin	**W:** 1-11
Wheat Products	**P:** 35
Whole-Grain Cereals	**A:** 45
Wine	**A:** 38; **E:** 8; **P:** 10; **S:** 51
Woodruff	**A:** 85

X

Xylose	**A:** 11; **C:** 44, 57, 64; **M:** 24; **N:** 11; **P:** 23, 41, 51

Y

Yeast	**P:** 35
Yogurt	**C:** 52

Z

Zafirlukast	**Z:** 1
Zalcitabine	**Z:** 2
Zidovudine	**Z:** 3
Zinc	**A:** 15; **C:** 52, 72; **D:** 3, 26, 36; **E:** 1, 17; **F:** 6, 19; **I:** 23; **M:** 27; **O:** 9; **P:** 5; **S:** 29; **T:** 3, 26; **V:** 6; **W:** 6; **Z:** 4, 6
Zolpidem	**Z:** 5